DR. N. AGGAr

# Aids to General Practice

*For Churchill Livingstone*

*Commissioning Editor:* Timothy Horne
*Copy Editor:* Isla MacLean
*Project Controllers:* Nancy Arnott, Kay Hunston

# Aids to General Practice

**Michael Mead**

BSc MB BS DCH DRCOG MRCGP
General Practitioner
Leicestershire

THIRD EDITION

CHURCHILL LIVINGSTONE
EDINBURGH HONG KONG LONDON MADRID MELBOURNE NEW YORK
AND TOKYO 1995

CHURCHILL LIVINGSTONE
Medical Division of Pearson Professional Limited

Distributed in the United States of America by
Churchill Livingstone Inc., 650 Avenue of the Americas,
New York, N.Y. 10011, and by associated companies,
branches and representatives throughout the world.

First edition 1988
Second edition 1990
Third edition 1995

ISBN 0 443 05277 8

**British Library Cataloguing in Publication Data**
A catalogue record for this book is available from
the British Library.

**Library of Congress Cataloging in Publication Data**
A catalog record for this book is available from the
Library of Congress.

The
publisher's
policy is to use
**paper manufactured
from sustainable forests**

Produced by Longman Singapore Publishers (Pte) Ltd
Printed in Singapore

# Contents

# Preface to the Third Edition

This book summarizes the essentials of general practice, in terms of both common clinical conditions and practice management. Written in the 'Aids' format of lists and tables, it will be particularly useful for trainees revising for the MRCGP exam and students sitting examinations or assessments as part of their undergraduate curriculum. All the everyday problems of a typical surgery are here – from otitis media to cystitis, from hypertension to prescribing the pill, from croup to backache. All aspects of prevention and screening are covered, and there are also chapters on prescribing and antenatal care. A trainee or young principal will thus find the contents both practical and highly relevant to their daily consultations. It is also hoped that the book will be valuable to students during their introductory attachments to general practice, when they are first exposed to the wide range of non-specific presentations presented to the family doctor – from a child with a recurrent cough to a patient who is habitually tired.

The large chapter on practice management will undoubtedly be welcomed by trainees and students as this area is often neglected in the medical literature. The sections on the GP's 1990 Contract, fundholding, medical records, the health care team, income, expenditure, visiting premises, etc., should be committed to memory by any candidate approaching the MRCGP.

This third edition sees much new material in both the clinical and practice management sections. Of major importance have been the British Thoracic Society's new guidelines on asthma and the appreciation of the role of *Helicobacter pylori* in the pathogenesis of peptic ulcers. Newer drugs (e.g. sumatriptan) and vaccines (e.g. Hib vaccine and HAVRIX) are furthering the advance of medicine. On the practice management front, the health promotion banding payments have appeared, as has a new system for handling complaints.

I am deeply indebted to the staff of Update and the publishers (Reed Healthcare Communications) for permission to publish some

of the tables in the Practice Management chapter, which first
appeared in the *Trainees' Guide to Practice Management* series in
issues of *Trainee*.

1995                                                    M.G.M.

# Medicine

## HYPERTENSION

Mortality and morbidity related to both systolic and diastolic BP, although most statistics relate to the diastolic BP

### Current guidelines
*In the under 65s*

| | |
|---|---|
| Diastolic BP < 90 mmHg | Normotensive |
| Diastolic BP 90–99 mmHg | Borderline to mild hypertension |
| Diastolic BP 100–109 mmHg | Moderate hypertension |
| Diastolic BP ⩾ 100 mmHg | Severe hypertension |

Systolic BP > 160 mmHg is raised in the under 65s and by itself is an indication for treatment, regardless of the diastolic blood pressure.

Therefore, raised BP is > 160/90 mmHg in the under 65s (although life insurance companies take > 140/90 mmHg).

*The elderly*
There is now good evidence that reduction of blood pressure in the elderly can reduce strokes and cardiovascular mortality (e.g. The European Working Party on High Blood Pressure in the Elderly Trial (Amery A et al 1985)), at least in the 60–80 age group. The current consensus of opinion is swinging towards treating hypertension in the elderly, although the benefits of treatment in the over 80 age group are less well defined and the side-effects of the drugs may be intolerable in this age group.

Most physicians would at least reduce therapy to a minimum in the over 80s and certainly regard a higher level of blood pressure as being acceptable. Aiming to drop the BP below 160/90 mmHg in the over 80s will inevitably lead to drug-related problems, including postural hypotension.

### Statistics
1. Only half the patients with significantly raised blood pressure are known to their doctors (more since the New Contract).

2. About 5% of your adult patients will have a diastolic BP of 110 mmHg or more, and a much larger percentage will have a diastolic BP between 90 and 110 mmHg
3. Around one-third of middle-aged patients will be classed in official terms as hypertensive

**Recording the BP**
1. Check sphygmomanometer and calibrate regularly
2. Use the appropriate cuff, i.e. larger cuffs for obese arms
3. Record with patient sitting relaxed after a few minutes, rest and the arm horizontal
4. Estimate systolic pressure by pressure required to stop brachial artery pulsation
5. Apply stethoscope over artery and inflate cuff to 30 mmHg above estimated systolic. Deflate cuff recording
   (i)  when sounds first appear (systolic)
   (ii) when sounds disappear (the diastolic or 5th Korotkoff sound)
   The point of muffling of sounds (4th Korotkoff sound) is recorded if sounds continue until zero
6. Record to the nearest 2 mmHg
7. Repeat recording after 2 or 3 min–if > 10 mmHg difference, take the best of three readings
8. If the diastolic BP is above 90 mmHg but less than 100 mmHg, the blood pressure should be measured three more times over a 3–6 month period–a decision to treat will depend on other risk factors. If the diastolic is 100–109 mmHg ask patient to return for a second reading in 2 weeks time and then 2 weeks after that for a third reading
   THE PATIENT'S BP ON WHICH A DECISION IS TO BE MADE MUST BE THE AVERAGE OF AT LEAST THREE READINGS TAKEN ON SEPARATE OCCASIONS, e.g.

| Date | BP (mmHg) |
|------|-----------|
| 1.10.86 | 166 |
|         | 102 |
| 14.10.86 | 162 |
|          | 110 |
| 28.10.86 | 158 |
|          | 106 |

Therefore, mean BP of patient = 162/106 mmHg

The purists would recommend a fourth reading after a further 2 weeks observation. If the BP is falling further, observation can be at monthly intervals. With a diastolic BP > 110 mmHg but < 130 mmHg one would like the three readings completed in 2 weeks. Severe hypertension (diastolic BP 130 mmHg and above) should be referred straight away without the three-reading rule and admission arranged if causing an encephalopathy, cardiac or renal failure.

## Screening for hypertension

1. Aim of every practice should be to record BP of every patient aged 15–74 years. This is a requirement of the health promotion banding system. To achieve this:
   (i) Record BP of every new patient at the New Registration Check (see later)
   (ii) For existing patients, two alternatives:
      a. Instituting a screening programme using the age – sex register to send appointments to patients and checking on attendance
      b. Adopting a 'case finding' approach whereby a sticker is put into the records of every patient over the age of 15 years reminding the doctor to check the BP at the next attendance (assuming it hasn't been checked in the last 3 years). Since 75% of patients consult their GP in a year and 95% within 5  years, this is an effective method
2. The BP of all patients should be checked every 3 years
3. Every practice should set up a register of its hypertensives – again a health promotion banding requirement

## Hypertension clinics

1. Increasingly being set up using practice nurses
2. They are in effect 'cardiovascular risk factor' clinics
3. Each patient should have their own follow-up card as shown in Table 1

## Risk factors

Target organ damage (retinopathy, proteinuria, raised urea and creatinine, cardiomegaly and ECG changes) indicates the worse prognosis in terms of risk. Family history is the next most important risk factor. Other risk factors include:
Young age ( < 45 years)
Being male
Diabetes mellitus
Raised serum cholesterol
Smoking
Obesity
Excess alcohol intake
High salt intake
Race
Stress
*Note*: Losing weight, stopping smoking, reducing alcohol and salt intake will all lower blood pressure

## Causes

1. In the general practice setting a vast majority (95% +) of hypertensives will be those with essential hypertension

**Table 1**   Example of what a hypertension card might look like

| NAME: | | | AGE: |
|---|---|---|---|
| | Date + BP | Date + BP | Date + BP |
| Initial BP Readings | 1. | 2. | 3. |
| Therefore mean BP initially = | | | |

EXAMINATION
Pulse:
Heart size:
Heart sounds:
Femoral pulses:
Chest:
Fundi:

INVESTIGATIONS
Urine:
Urea and electrolytes:
Creatinine:
Lipids:

RISK FACTORS
Weight, Body mass index =
Smoking
Family history hypertension/ischaemic heart disease
Hyperlipidaemia
Diabetes mellitus

CURRENT DRUG                    NEXT REVIEW DATE:
THERAPY AND DATE:

2. Make sure patient is not on the pill or steroids
3. Check femoral pulses in younger patients and that the patient is
   not Cushingoid
4. Renal disease should be looked for – test urine and order urea,
   electrolytes and creatinine in all hypertensive patients
5. Listening for renal artery bruits is beyond the average GP
   and without history of palpitations, sweating or marked
   fluctuation in BP, screening for phaeochromocytoma is not
   indicated

**Investigation**
Apart from the above a CXR for cardiomegaly and an ECG for
left ventricular hypertrophy (LVH) may be appropriate for
moderate hypertensives or where there is a suggestion of
LVH or cardiac failure, but hardly appropriate for all
hypertensives.

**Referral**
1. Those with renal disease or other causes of hypertension
2. Those with labile BP

3. Those with severe hypertension
4. Those not controlled by your therapy
5. The young (< 35 years)

**MRC trial on mild hypertension**
1. Over 17 000 patients were studied in 190 general practices
2. Patients were mild hypertensives DBP 90–109 mmHg, aged 35–64 years
3. Target of treatment was to lower DBP to 90 mmHg
4. Treatment was with either bendrofluazide or propranolol
5. Results MRC Working Party 1985 include:
    (i) If 850 mild hypertensives are treated for 1 year, about one stroke will be prevented
   (ii) Treatment makes no difference to mortality rate or to rate of coronary events
  (iii) Difference between smokers and non-smokers for stroke is greater than the effect of antihypertensive therapy (again emphasizing a 'risk factor' approach)

**Suggested management**
1. For those with BP < 160/90 mmHg repeat in 3 years
2. For those with a diastolic BP of 90 mmHg or over on three separate readings, complete the examination and investigations on the follow-up card and advise on any risk factors (including reducing alcohol and salt intake)
3. The management protocol shown in Table 2 would seem reasonable considering the current guidelines

**Suggested treatment protocol for hypertension**
Aim is diastolic BP at 90 mmHg and systolic BP 160 mmHg, i.e. < 160/90 mmHg

*Young (< 65 years)*
1. First choice a β-blocker, e.g. atenolol but if asthmatic, cardiac failure, peripheral vascular disease/Raynaud's or problems with side-effects of β-blocker, start an ACE inhibitor or calcium antagonist. ACE inhibitors first choice in diabetics.
2. If control not achieved, i.e. diastolic > 90 mmHg, then add thiazide diuretic to β-blocker or add calcium antagonist to β-blocker or thiazide to calcium antagonist or increase the dose of ACE inhibitor
3. If still no control, then try triple therapy with thiazide diuretic + β-blocker (providing no contraindications) + vasodilator e.g. nifedipine or add to the ACE inhibitor

**Table 2**   Management protocol

| Diastolic BP 90–94 mmHg | Diastolic BP 95–99 mmHg | Diastolic BP 100–104 mmHg | Diastolic BP 105–129 mmHg | Diastolic BP 130+ mmHg |
|---|---|---|---|---|
| Advice on weight, smoking, alcohol and salt intake | Advice on weight, smoking, alcohol and salt intake | Despite MRC trial it is still probably wise to treat all those with a sustained DBP of 100 mmHg or over, especially if there is any other risk factor | Treat all | Refer |
| Check at 6 months, 1 year, then yearly. Consider treatment in those with major risk factors | Treat those with major risk factors (young males, poor family history, etc.). Those not treated should be followed regularly every 3 months | | | Malignant hypertension with visual symptoms or symptoms of cardiac or renal failure needs urgent admission |

*Notes:*
1. A systolic BP > 160 mmHg also merits treatment independently of the diastolic pressure
2. As noted previously, the elderly will also benefit from treatment in the treatable groups, at least until 80 years old when the treatment might be reviewed
3. With all patients, particularly those not in the treatment group, stress non-drug ways of reducing blood pressure viz:
   (i)   Losing weight (if obese)
   (ii)  Reducing alcohol intake
   (iii) Reducing salt intake
   (iv)  Stopping smoking

*Elderly (> 65 years)]*
1. Thiazide diuretic, e.g. 2.5 mg of bendrofluazide but not if diabetes or gout. As an alternative consider a calcium antagonist. With normal diet should be no problems with potassium depletion, but check potassium levels if diet poor or on digoxin
2. If no response, try thiazide diuretic + calcium antagonist (β-blockers often poorly tolerated in elderly)
3. If still no response, may be worth considering an ACE inhibitor or β-blocker therapy. A question of judging control versus side-effects

*Notes:*
1. If these regimes fail and compliance is good, then refer
2. ACE inhibitors have several uses:
    (i) Hypertension treatment, especially for those intolerant of β-blockers or with raised lipids (β-blockers have an adverse effect on lipids)
    (ii) Heart failure treatment
    (iii) Preventing development of diabetic nephropathy – may be agents of choice here
    (iv) For those with poor myocardial function after a myocardial infarction

Note that diuretics should be stopped 48 h prior to ACE inhibitor therapy for hypertension, the initial dose should be given with the patient supire at night and the urea/creatinine and electrolyte levels should be checked before and 2 weeks after treatment – if there is deterioration in renal function, stop the drug and investigate for renal artery stenosis. About 20% of patients develop a cough with ACE inhibitors

## PREVENTION OF CORONARY HEART DISEASE (CHD)

Most GPs now run preventive clinics and screening programmes looking for risk factors associated with the development of CHD as part of their health promotion programme. The risk factors are:
Smoking
Hypertension
Diabetes mellitus
High blood lipids
Family history of CHD
Obesity
Excess alcohol consumption (effect on lipids and weight)
Oral contraceptive pill
Type A personality (competitive, aggressive, impatient)

? Stress
? Lack of exercise
? High salt intake
Males more at risk. Most of the above are covered elsewhere in the book.

## HYPERLIPIDAEMIA

1. Hypercholesterolaemia is principal risk factor but hypertriglyceridaemia is also a risk
2. Guidelines for screening for lipids are:
   (i) Screen particularly those with history or family history of CHD, with tendon xanthomata or a corneal arcus, with hypertension or diabetes or with a family history of hyperlipidaemia
   (ii) Limit to those below 65 years
   (iii) Refer those with true familial hypercholesterolaemia who are most at risk – may need drugs and certainly need close
   (iv) A random blood test is sufficient, as an initial screen for hyperlipidaemia monitoring
   (v) Regarding serum cholesterol
   < 5 mmol/l is normal
   5–6.5 mmol/l requires dietary advice although drug treatment might be considered for a patient with existing CHD (e.g. has had a bypass graft) or major risk factors.
   6.5–7.8 mmol/l may require drug therapy in addition to diet. A fasting cholesterol and an HDL cholesterol and triglycerides should be measured and secondary causes of hyperlipidaemia (hypothyroidism, diabetes, excess alcohol intake, renal or hepatic failure) excluded. Start a lipid-lowering diet and recheck lipids in 3 months. If diet fails despite compliance and the patients has other risk factors (an HDL cholesterol < 0.9 mmol/l, family or personal history of coronary artery disease, hypertension, etc.), drugs should be considered.
   > 7.8 mmol/l will probably require drug therapy in addition to diet. Repeat on a fasting sample, exclude secondary causes and refer to a dietition. If diet fails after 6 months, treat irrespective of other risk factors. If the cholesterol is > 9 mmol/l refer to your local lipid clinic
   (vi) Drug therapy
      a. For mild hypercholesterolaemia alone the first choice is either cholestyramine (Questran) or colestipol (Colestid), reserving simvastatin (Zocor) or pravastatin (Lipostat) for patients with moderate or severe hypercholesterolaemia or if the resins fail or are

unpalatable. If the triglycerides and cholesterol are raised, the first-line treatment is a fibrate e.g. gemfibrizol (Lopid), bezafibrate (Bezalip), fenofibrate (Lipantyl) or ciprofibrate (Modalim)

b Before prescribing lipid-lowering agents read their specific drug interactions, contraindications, side-effects and suggested monitoring programmes (i.e. measuring liver function tests/muscle enzymes as well as lipid levels)

## MYOCARDIAL INFARCTION (MI)

Nearly one-half of patients die with a myocardial infarction and one-third die from ventricular fibrillation prior to hospital admission

### Treatment of an acute infarct

1. For pain, diamorphine 5 mg i.v. (with 2.5 mg i.v. at 10-min intervals, as required) plus prochlorperazine (Stemetil). Alternatively use Cyclimorph 10 mg i.v.
2. For left ventricular failure (LVF) i.v. frusemide and for bradycardia (< 50/min) atropine (starting with 0.3 mg i.v.)
3. A Nitrolingual spray is useful in the acute management and all patients (unless sensitive to aspirin or it is contraindicated) should be given a stat dose of 300 mg of aspirin, which has been shown to increase survival
4. Preventable deaths largely from ventricular fibrillation in the first few hours – portable defibrillators carried by GPs would help. Recent studies on the administration of antiarrhythmics to treat ventricular fibrillation have shown that these agents are ineffective in the acute stage
5. Since cardiac arrest is sudden, a major contribution to saving lives would be to train everyone in the art of cardiopulmonary resuscitation (CPR)
6. It has been shown that the use of i.v. streptokinase can reduce mortality if given in the acute stage of a myocardial infarction preferably within an hour of onset. After 12 h benefit is less certain. Antistreplase (Eminase), which is given slowly i.v. over 4–5 min, has been used by GPs a long distance from hospital, e.g. in rural Scotland

### Home versus hospital

With current advances in thrombolytic and anti-arrhythmic therapy the pendulum has swung firmly to urgent hospital admission for all patients

**Rehabilitation and prevention**
1. Mobilize early – aim for 2 months before resuming work and sexual activity
2. DVLC must be informed – normal driving permitted after 2 months but patient may not be allowed to drive an LGV or PCV
3. Certain β-blockers have been shown to prevent re-infarction and reduce mortality when given after an infarct e.g. propranolol, atenolol, metoprolol and timolol. Aspirin has also been shown to be beneficial post-infarction
4. ACE inhibitors are now increasingly used post infarct for those with impaired left ventricular function

*Note*: With the advent of angioplasty and coronary artery bypass grafts it is increasingly the responsibility of the GP to refer younger patients with ischaemic heart disease to cardiologists for full assessment, exercise testing, coronary angiography, etc.

## MANAGEMENT OF THE DIABETIC PATIENT IN GENERAL PRACTICE

1. Diabetic care programmes are financially rewarded as part of health promotion payments (see page 148 for further details)
2. All practice nurses looking after the care of diabetics should fully trained and a care system should be evolved dividing responsibility between nurse and doctor. Remember fundoscopy!

**Initial interview with a new diabetic joining the practice**
1. Are they under the hospital?
2. What drugs/insulin dose are they on? Do they fully understand their therapy?
3. Check on patient's monitoring – urine tests and/or blood tests
4. What is the current control like? (? hypoglycaemic episodes, ? any recent changes in therapy, ? recent urine or blood results, ? complications)
5. Education
    (i) General understanding of diabetes (not to stop insulin if ill, when to call a doctor, etc.)
    (ii) Understanding of the need for follow-up
    (iii) Diet
    (iv) Smoking
6. When did the patient last have an 'official' check-up? (blood sugar, glycosylated haemoglobin, etc.)
7. Organize a follow-up plan

**Suggested follow-up**
1.  Every 6 months:
    - (i)  Review patient's own monitoring
    - (ii)  Blood sugar with glucometer. A random blood glucose < 10 mmol/l is the aim
    - (iii)  Weigh and discuss diet
    - (iv)  Test urine for glucose and protein
    - (v)  Glycosylated haemoglobin – this gives a measure of the average blood sugar levels over the previous 6–10 weeks and is currently the most useful method of monitoring diabetic control
      Normal range: 5–9%
      Aim for < 10%. Over is unacceptable
    - (vi)  Ask patient if there are any particular problems
    - (vii)  Check on injection sites
2.  Annually:
    - (i)  Check feet:
      - a.  peripheral pulses? ischaemia
      - b.  Sensation and reflexes
      - c.  Any evidence of infection?
    - (ii)  General examination, especially of the cardiovascular system
    - (iii)  Blood pressure
    - (iv)  Urea and electrolytes, creatinine and fasting lipids
    - (v)  Mid-stream urine
    - (vi)  Examination of fundi and visual acuity, although many would say this should be 6-monthly. Early diagnosis and treatment (laser photocoagulation) of retinopathy can prevent blindness. If not experienced at fundoscopy, arrange regular ophthalmological assessment at the hospital, especially for young insulin-dependent diabetics

Newly diagnosed diabetics will clearly need to be seen more frequently. Just as with hypertension try and use a special follow-up card.

**Diagnosis of diabetes**
A fasting blood glucose > 8 mmol/l or a random blood glucose > 11 mmol/l

**Notes on diabetes**
1.  Diabetic Health Visitor invaluable source of support, education and monitoring. Management of diabetics should be a team approach
2.  For hypoglycaemia in diabetics glucagon i.m. very useful
3.  Most accurate monitoring is by blood test, e.g. using BM stix

(prescribable by GPs). May be that patients should have their own glucometers, if they can use them
4. If at all interested in diabetes or setting up your own mini-clinic, the RCGP have produced a folder on diabetes that contains all the information you need PLUS sample co-op and follow-up cards. Purchase a copy!

## MANAGEMENT OF THE EPILEPTIC PATIENT IN GENERAL PRACTICE

### Acute attack
1. For febrile convulsions *see* Paediatric chapter
2. For a *grand mal* convulsion, diazepam 10 mg i.v. slowly, repeated as necessary. Remember to protect the airway

### Referral
1. For febrile convulsions *see* Paediatric chapter
2. For a *grand mal* convulsion I would refer at the first seizure for full investigation and assessment. Particularly beware first onset of epilepsy over 25 years old, as idiopathic epilepsy rare after this age

### Long-term management of the established epileptic
1. Ensure the diagnosis has been firmly established – especially with older patients who may have been labelled 'epileptic' on dubious criteria.
2. Aim for an annual review. Epileptics often not followed up and end up with long-term repeat prescriptions. May wish to set up a register
3. Assess the drug therapy
   (i) Is the drug at the correct dose and frequency?
   (ii) Are fits being controlled?
   (iii) After 3 fit-free years, phased withdrawal of the drugs may be worthwhile in some patients but beware if patient drives as another fit will prejudice their licence and you will not be popular!
4. Monitor and adjust the therapy as appropriate
   (i) Serum levels useful if fits not suppressed, signs of toxicity or non-compliance suspected
   (ii) Remember to test full blood count, calcium, alkaline phosphatase and liver function tests (especially in the early days of valproate treatment). Check about every 3 years
   (iii) Aim for simplest regime possible – preferably with one drug
   (iv) Watch out for side-effects/drug interactions

5. Support and help the epileptic
   (i) By discussion of employment, marital, driving and
       contraceptive problems
   (ii) By information about local self-help groups

**Driving and epilepsy**
1. Obtain a recent copy of *Medical Aspects of Fitness to
   Drive**
2. Current regulations[†] are:
   Epileptic may be granted a licence if controlled and
   (i) They have been free from an epileptic attack for
       1 year preceding the date when the licence is to have
       effect
   (ii) If attacks occur while asleep, they should have had attacks
        only while asleep at least 3 years prior to the granting of a
        licence

The proviso is that the patient would be safe driving in other
respects too, i.e. not a source of danger due to a cerebral
disorder, drug side-effects, etc. Note you cannot hold an
LGV or PCV licence if you have a liability to epileptic seizures.
For a single fit, consult above booklet regarding
regulation

## MANAGEMENT OF THE ASTHMATIC PATIENT IN GENERAL PRACTICE

Asthma is common (5% of adults, 10% of children) and can be fatal
(about 1500 deaths in Britain each year). *See also* Paediatric
chapter

**Acute attacks**
1. More often underestimated than overestimated
2. Use steroids early (underuse associated with unnecessary
   deaths)
3. For adults, standard treatment (assuming, of course,
   unresponsive to inhaled bronchodilators) is:
   High-dose inhaled β-agonist e.g. by nebulizer or, if not
   available, by spacer, plus systemic steroids (30–60 mg of
   prednisolone). If life-threatening features (PEF < 33% of
   predicted, exhaustion, bradycardia, cyanosis, silent chest)
   give i.v. aminophylline 250 mg by slow injection if not already

*Medical Commission on Accident Prevention, 35–43 Lincoln's Inn Fields,
London WC2A 3PN
[†]1982 Road Traffic Act, Motor Vehicles (Drivers Licences), Amendment No. 3

taking xanthines or $\beta_2$ stimulants by injection e.g. Ventolin 500 mg s.c. or Ventolin 250 mg in 5 ml by slow intravenous injection.
4. Hospital admission for severe attacks [tachycardia > 110/min, exhaustion, severe dyspnoea, quiet breath sounds (silent chest), marked accessory muscle respiration, peak expiratory flow rate < 50% of predicted value. Give steroids as above prior to admission
5. Nebulized salbutamol useful for children in attacks – some hospitals have open access. Problem with nebulizer use at home is excessive reliance on nebulizer and consequent underestimation of the attack and failure to call medical advice. Nevertheless nebulizers worth considering in general practice and to save admission to hospital – make sure patients understand their use and do not fail to call if nebuliser not relieving symptoms
6. For minor attacks simple $\beta_2$ stimulant preparations may suffice. If steroids used for acute attack, obviously follow up with an oral course

**Long-term management**
1. History from patient: assess severity, variability and precipitating factors
   (i) Family history
   (ii) Length of history of asthma – when first diagnosed
   (iii) Relation to exercise and work
   (iv) Search for allergens – RAST test in children and young adults. Also search for precipitating factors (salicylates, tartrazines in food, etc.)
   (v) Diurnal variation – ? morning dips
   (vi) Frequency of attacks and hospital admissions
   (vii) Time off work or school due to asthma
   (viii) May be useful to have a card for each patient listing history, allergens (results of RAST or skin tests), medication past and present and recorded PEFRs
   (ix) Grade into mild, moderate and severe according to the ten criteria listed in Table 3. Severe asthmatics must be monitored to check on progress, should be known to all in the practice and ideally should have open access to hospital
2. Education of the patient
   (i) Explain asthma (+ booklet)
   (ii) With childhood asthma advise on measures to counter the house-dust mite
   (iii) Demonstrate and check patient's techniques of using their inhalation system

**Table 3**    Criteria used to grade asthma

| | Mild asthma | Moderate asthma | Severe asthma |
|---|---|---|---|
| 1. Frequency of attacks | Few | Occasional | Frequent |
| 2. Time off school/work | Nil | Occasional day | Often |
| 3. Acute hospital admissions | Nil | Nil | Yes |
| 4. Restriction of daily activity | Nil | Rarely | Limited |
| 5. Diurnal variation | Little | Slight variation | Disturbed sleep due to early morning dips |
| 6. Bronchodilator usage | Occasional as required | More regularly | Virtually continuously – beware excessive use |
| 7. Other therapy | Nil | Intal or Becotide perhaps as prophylactic | Yes. Various preparations used |
| 8. Use of oral steroids | Never | Once or twice in the past as short courses | Several times. May be on regular oral steroids |
| 9. PEFR | May be near normal, especially between attacks, but in any case > 70% of predicted value | Variable | Sometimes drops to quite low levels, e.g. 200 l/min or less |
| 10. Patient's viewpoint | Hardly ever thinks about it. A mild nuisance | Occasional restriction. Keeps inhaler handy and may use prophylactic regularly | May have to plan life around asthma |

(iv) Check patient's understanding of when and now to use their medication and especially use of Ventolin before Becotide, if both inhalers used

(v) Encourage to stop smoking
(vi) Give guidelines on when to call a doctor (getting worse despite using inhalers, bad night, dyspnoeic, difficulty in speaking due to the breathing, etc.). Give severe asthmatics a spare supply of steroid (although still need to see a doctor) and make sure they do not run out
3. Monitoring of the patient
  (i) The PEFR is to the asthmatic what the BP is to the hypertensive
  (ii) Patients should have their own peak flow meter (can be prescribed)
  (iii) Normal values are about 500–600 l/min for adult men and 400–500 l/min for adult women
  (iv) Patients should record their own PEFR, especially if in the moderate group and essentially if severe. The record will
    a. Help plan therapy
    b. Detect diurnal variation (in chronic asthma > 20%), e.g. recorded at 500 l/min in afternoon but 180 l/min at 2 a.m.
    c. Indicate the severity of the attack. Patients daily record will be the baseline – if PEFR falls by more than half, the attack is severe
    d. Allow you to judge success of therapy
4. Adapting the treatment to the patient
  (i) Test reversibility by response to bronchodilators (PEFR should increase by at least 15%)
  (ii) Adapt delivery system to patient
    a. Children can use a Rotahaler or Spinhaler from about 4 years and by 7 years most can manage an inhaler
    b. Spacing devices, e.g. Volumatic for Ventolin help those with poor technique
  (iii) All patients should have a self-management plan
  (iv) Therapy for asthma should follow the 1993 guidelines of the British Thoracic Society, published in *Thorax* (March 1993, Vol 48). Patients start treatment at the step appropriate to their condition. The guidelines, in condensed form, are:

## MANAGEMENT OF CHRONIC ASTHMA IN ADULTS

*Step 1*: OCCASIONAL USE OF RELIEF BRONCHODILATORS
In haled short-acting β-agonists for symptom relief. Check compliance and technique
*Step 2*: REGULAR INHALED ANTI-INFLAMMATORY AGENTS
Inhaled short-acting β-agonists as required plus beclomethasone or budesonide 100–400 mg twice daily
*Step 3*: HIGH-DOSE INHALED STEROIDS
Inhaled short-acting β-agonists as required plus beclomethasone or

budesonide increased to 800–2000 mg daily via a large volume spacer

*Step 4*: HIGH-DOSE INHALED STEROIDS AND REGULAR BRONCHODILATORS

As Step 3 plus a sequential trial of one or more of:
- Inhaled long-acting β-agonists (e.g. Serevent)
- Sustained–release theophylline
- Inhaled ipratropium or oxitropium
- Long-acting β-agonist tablets
- High-dose inhaled bronchodilators
- Cromoglycate or nedocromil

*Step 5*: ADDITION OF REGULAR STEROID TABLETS

Inhaled short-acting β-agonists as required with inhaled beclomethasone or budesonide (800–2000 mg daily via a large volume spacer) and one or more of the long-acting bronchodilators plus regular prednisolone tablets in a single daily dose

## MANAGEMENT OF CHRONIC ASTHMA IN CHILDREN

*Step 1*: OCCASIONAL USE OF RELIEF BRONCHODILATORS

Short-acting β-agonists as required

*Step 2*: REGULAR INHALED ANTI-INFLAMMATORY AGENTS

Intermittent short-acting β-agonist as required plus cromoglycote (Intal) as powder (20 mg thrice daily) or via metered dose inhaler and large volume spacer (10 mg thrice daily)

*Step 3*: INHALED STEROIDS

Inhaled short-acting β-agonists as required plus beclomethasone or budesonide 50–200 mg twice daily. Consider a 5-day course of soluble prednisolone 1–2 mg/kg/day or a temporary increase in inhaled steroids (double dose) for stabilization

*Step 4*: HIGH-DOSE INHALED STEROIDS

Inhaled short-acting β-agonists as required plus beclomethasone or budesonide increased to 400–800 mg via a large spacer or dry powder device. Consider short prednisolone course. Consider adding regular, twice daily long-acting β-agonist (Serevent can be used for children over 4 years)

*Step 5*:
a. HIGH DOSE INHALED STEROIDS AND BRONCHODILATORS
   Inhaled steroids 800 mg daily (treatment as Step 4) plus slow release xanthines or nebulized β-agonists
b. ADDITION OF REGULAR STEROIDS
   As in step 5a with the addition of alternate low-dose (5–10 mg) prednisolone

**Notes on treatment**
- Aim should be for minimal symptoms, a PEFR 80% of predicted or best and a circadian variation in peak flow of < 20%

- May be able to step down at 3–6 month treatment reviews
- Fluticasone (Flixotide) launched recently. It has:
  A low bio availability (i.e. negligible systemic effect)
  A weight-for-weight potency twice that of beclomethasone
  (Becotide)
  It is licensed for children over 4 years of age
- Little substantiated evidence of inhaled steroids significantly
  suppressing growth in childhood

## COUGH

Commonest presenting symptom in general practice

### Causes
1. Upper respiratory tract infection – as part of a coryzal illness, laryngitis, etc.
2. Lower respiratory tract infection – including croup, bronchitis, pneumonia, etc.
3. Other specific infections involving the respiratory tract, e.g. tuberculosis, measles
4. Diseases involving the lungs, e.g. fibrosing alveolitis, cystic fibrosis
5. Carcinoma of the lung
6. Inhaled foreign body
7. Asthma
8. Left ventricular failure with pulmonary oedema
9. Smoking

### Notes
1. For cough in children *see* Paediatric chapter
2. A persistent cough in an older person may be the sign of more serious disease – especially carcinoma of the lung in a smoker. Remember also left ventricular failure as a cause of cough in the elderly and late-onset asthma
3. As a general rule, a cough persisting greater than 3 weeks or associated with other symptoms, e.g. dyspnoea, haemoptysis, etc., merits more serious consideration

### Management
1. Depends on diagnosis – bronchodilators/steroids for asthma, diuretics for LVF, antibiotics for pneumonia, etc.
2. Vast majority will be simple respiratory infections. Approach can be:
   (i) Advice – simple inhalations, aspirin, stop smoking, etc.
   (ii) Advice plus antibiotic
       Criteria for an antibiotic might be:

a. Presence of chest signs (crepitations, bronchial breathing, etc.)
b. Infective exacerbation of asthma or chronic bronchitis
c. Patient ill (pyrexia, etc.)
d. Prolonged infection (> 3 weeks)
e. High-risk groups, e.g. elderly, those with other disease

(iii) Prescription of, or advice to purchase, a cough medicine
a. Not useful if cough productive of sputum or a reflection of asthma
b. May be useful for a dry cough serving no purpose
c. Choice of cough medicine
Mild cough: simple linctus
Moderate cough: codeine or pholcodine linctus
Cough in terminal illness: methadone linctus
d. Problems of cough medicines include constipation and dependence with the opiate preparations (e.g. codeine linctus), an excess of sugar detrimental to diabetics (but there are sugar-free linctuses), and sedative and sympathomimetic effects of some combination mixtures

## CHRONIC BRONCHITIS
Cough every day with sputum for 3 months a year, for at least 2 consecutive years

**Management**
1. Full assessment
   (i) Any evidence of heart failure? e.g. ankle oedema, raised JVP
   (ii) Differentiate from late onset asthma (no history of smoking, wheezy in attacks, PMH of hay fever and eczema, reversibility of airways as shown by a trial of steroids or bronchodilators)
   (iii) Has there been any recent deterioration, haemoptysis or weight loss? (Consider in these instances a CXR to exclude a neoplasm)
   (iv) What degree of emphysema is present, if any?
   (v) How much does the chronic bronchitis interfere with the patient's life?
   (vi) Full blood count (? anaemia contributing to symptoms or a secondary polycythaemia) and a PEFR (reversible airways obstruction should be demonstrated)
2. Advice
   (i) Stop smoking
   (ii) Lose weight if overweight

    (iii)  Contact the GP if worsening dyspnoea, purulent sputum, haemoptysis or weight loss

    (iv)  Maintain a reserve supply of antibiotics at home

    (v)  Consider influenza vaccination in the autumn

3. Treatment

  Acute exacerbations:

    (i)  Usual organisms are *Haemophilus influenzae* and *Streptococcus pneumoniae*. Antibiotic most useful is amoxycillin

    (ii)  Bronchodilators – worth a try, e.g. salbutamol by the various inhalational systems

    (iii)  Short course of steroids for 10 days if no contraindications and the situation merits the trial

    (iv)  Avoid sedative drugs and hypnotics

    (v)  Treat heart failure, e.g. with Frumil. Digoxin useful if in atrial fibrillation

    (vi)  Inhaled steam useful for loosening secretions

## Chronic management

1. Advice as above plus a spare course of antibiotics
2. Help at home, e.g. rehousing if damp conditions, home help, meals-on-wheels
3. Education about use of drugs. The following may be useful:
   - (i) $\beta_2$ stimulants, e.g. salbutamol (Ventolin)
   - (ii) Oral theophyllines,
   - (iii) Ipratropium bromide (Atrovent inhaler) – a useful preparation in chronic bronchitis, which can profitably be combined withe the use of a $\beta_2$ stimulant inhaler, i.e. they should be used concurrently
   - (iv) Diuretics if heart failure present
   - (v) Steroids – preferably inhaled but only if necessary and their efficiency (i.e. bronchodilation) has been documented in the given patient
4. Some patients can be instructed in physiotherapy, postural drainage, etc.
5. Domiciliary oxygen. Can reduce mortality in chronic bronchitics but to be effective must be given for 15 h/day, i.e. virtually continuously. Best method in general practice is by using an oxygen concentrator. If cylinders are used it is essential
   - (i) That the patient can use them properly
   - (ii) Concentrations no higher than 24–28% are used, so that the hypoxic drive is not diminished

## Notes

1. Mucolytics generally unhelpful
2. Avoid cough medicines containing respiratory depressants, i.e. opiates

**SMOKING**

Single most preventable cause of ill health
GP can help by:
1. Mentioning it when patient presents with a smoking-related illness (e.g. cough) for follow-up of hypertension, contraception, etc.
2. Making a note in the records, to remind in the future
3. Helping the particular patient to give up by
    (i) Stressing the benefits in a friendly rather than condemnatory manner
    (ii) Providing a booklet, e.g. *Give up smoking**
    (iii) Discussing some of the difficulties in giving up smoking
    (iv) Advising, in conjunction with the practice nurse on the benefits of using nicotine patches or chewing gum

**HAY FEVER**

Symptoms of rhinorrhoea, sneezing, conjunctivitis and sometimes wheeze, starting in late May and lasting through June and July

**Treatment**
1. For eye symptoms: Opticrom
2. For nasal symptoms: Beconase, Flixonase or Syntaris nasal spray. The steroid nasal sprays, if used sparingly and sensibly, seem more effective for patients in the season than using regular cromoglycate (Rynacrom)
3. Antihistamines: e.g. terfenadine (Triludan)
*Note*: For severe hay fever, or approaching exams, a course of oral steroids is a reasonable course of action (provided no contraindications). Depot steroid injections (e.g. Kenalog) are used by some but beware adrenal suppression and muscle wasting at the site of injection. Kenalog should be given by deep i.m. injection into the gluteal muscle

**Desensitization**
Since 1980, 11 patients have died from severe anaphylactic reactions following treatment with desensitizing vaccines.[†] The CSMs (1986) recommendation that full resuscitation facilities be available has effectively ended their use in general practice, regardless of the pros and cons.

*Published by Action on Smoking and Health (5–11) Mortimer Street, London,
†Committee Safety Medicines (CSM), October 1986

## HEADACHE

Apart from the acute headache associated with a viral illness or sinusitis, by far the commonest causes of headache in general practice are tension headaches and migraine. Other causes apart from these are:
1. Sudden onset
   (i) Meningitis
   (ii) Cerebral haemorrhage, including subarachnoid haemorrhage
   (iii) Glaucoma
   (iv) Severe hypertension with hypertensive encephalopathy
2. Subacute
   (i) Post-traumatic headache. (NB Beware a developing subdural haematoma)
   (ii) Temporal arteritis
   (iii) Brain tumour
3. Chronic: cervical spondylosis

### Notes on the diagnosis of headache
1. Take care with the history – separate the acute from the recurrent, chronic headaches
2. Beware acute severe headache, especially with no previous history
3. Ask about associated symptoms (visual, nausea, etc.), site of headache, aggravating and relieving factors
4. Beware headaches in the elderly – remember temporal arteritis
5. While headache is not a common symptom of hypertension, it is wise to check the BP – the patient will expect it!
6. Ask the patient what he or she feels is the cause – it may be that a friend or relative has recently had a stroke or brain tumour. Reassurance may be all that is required
7. The headache of raised intracranial pressure typically occurs in the morning and is initially intermittent. Later it begins to wake the patient in the morning and may be associated with vomiting
8. As a general rule histories of headache > 6 months are extremely unlikely to be due to a malignant brain tumour – the course is much shorter
9. Beware 'migraine' presenting for the first time in a patient over 40 years – unusual to occur de novo in middle age

## MIGRAINE

Try and make a positive diagnosis
Migraine is:
1. Episodic headache, lasting for 4–72 hours with freedom between attacks

2. Commonly unilateral but not always the same side
3. Usually associated with gastrointestinal symptoms (anorexia, nausea, vomiting)
4. Sometimes preceded by a visual, sensory or motor aura (only one-fifth of patients)
5. Often familial

Tension headaches, on the other hand, tend to be a continuous generalized headache with no gastrointestinal or neurological symptoms, and occurring every day without relief. Ask about stress in the patient's life and look out for an underlying depression (early morning waking, etc.)

**Trigger factors for migraine**
Fatigue
Anxiety, stress, depression
Diet – fasting, irregular meals, certain foods (e.g. cheese and chocolate)
Alcohol
Flickering lights
Smoking
Change in lifestyle – travelling, new job, etc.
The contraceptive pill and other hormonal changes (menopause, menstruation, premenstrual)

**Treatment of an acute attack**
1. Treatment of choice for the mild attack is either paracetamol or aspirin, preferably in effervescent form
2. Gastric stasis and vomiting impair absorption so that metoclopramide (Maxolon) should be given a few minutes before the paracetamol or aspirin, either orally or i.m. Metoclopramide is combined with paracetamol in Paramax sachets
3. Metoclopramide plus analgesia should be all that is required in the mild cases (plus avoidance of trigger factors). NSAIDs can be more effective but watch for GI side-effects. Ergotamine should not now be prescribed – addiction and overdose is a danger and ironically one of the signs of habitual use is an 'ergotamine headache'. If simple analgesia or NSAID, fail, use sumatriptan (Imigran) –
   A selective 5HT agonist: > 70% successful in acute attacks'.
   Can be given at any stage in the attack (but advise early use)
   Relieves also the associated GI symptoms
   Comes in oral and injectable form (which is faster-acting)
   Contraindications include uncontrolled hypertension, ischaemic heart disease, previous myocardial infarction, Prinzmetal's angina, concomitant use of ergotamine, use of MAOIs, 5HT reuptake inhibitors and lithium

**Prophylaxis**

For recurrent migraine, e.g. more than two disabling attacks a month:

1. First choice in general practice should probably be a β-blocker, providing no contraindications – propranolol the first choice, e.g. Half Inderal LA
2. Pizotifen (Sanomigran), e.g. 1.5 mg nocte but side-effects (drowsiness, anticholinergic effects, weight gain, etc.) often mitigate against continuing the therapy
3. Recently, regular naproxen (Synflex, Naprosyn) has been shown to be a prophylaxis for migraine
4. Antidepressants or tranquillizers have their role to play in specific patients, e.g. amitriptyline 25 mg nocte which is effective over and above its use as an antidepressant.
5. Regular aspirin (providing no contraindications) also effective

*Note*: Methysergide use is best restricted to hospital but it is still a very useful drug in prophylaxis, if the above fail

## CYSTITIS

Better term is the 'frequency and dysuria syndrome'

**Notes**
1. Only 50% of women with dysuria and frequency will have significant bacteriuria
2. Some presenting with 'cystitis' will, in fact, have a vaginitis. Vulval inflammation due to *Candida* can cause 'cystitis' and *Trichomonas* can cause dysuria
3. In postmenopausal women an atrophic urethritis may respond to oestrogens
4. Recently established that some 'negative' cultures are due to infection with less easily grown microorganisms, e.g. *Chlamydia* and lactobacilli

**Management**
1. In adults, attacks of cystitis, even with a proven UTI, have never been shown to lead to hypertension or renal failure, hence an MSU in every case is pointless – although it is important to document and thoroughly treat UTI in pregnancy
2. For an acute attack:
   (i) Advise a high fluid intake and frequent voiding
   (ii) Short courses of antibiotics (3-day or even single-dose) are now used in the majority of patients. Only about 50% of pathogens are now sensitive to amoxycillin – trimethoprim is the current first-choice treatment. Traditional 7-day courses should still be used in men, pregnant women, diabetics, immunosuppressed patients, patients with renal

pain, renal tenderness, gross haematuria, renal disease and any abnormality of the urinary tract (see reference by Kay and Bailie). 75% of cases of bacterial UTI are due to *Escherichia coli*

(iii) Alkalizing agents will give symptomatic relief

3. For recurrent frequency and dysuria:
   (i) MSUs are useful – to document infection as the cause and determine the sensitivities
   (ii) Consider the precipitating factors of recurrent dysuria and frequency viz:
   Cold weather
   Psychological stress
   The menopause (i.e. oestrogen deficiency)
   Menstruation
   Sexual intercourse
   Sensitivity to locally used deodorants and antiseptics
   (iii) Advice
      a. If associated with sexual intercourse:
         Void after intercourse
         Use lubricants, e.g. KY jelly to lessen trauma
         Wash before and after intercourse
         Try a single dose of nitrofurantoin 50 mg after intercourse
      b. Maintain good perineal hygiene, washing from the front backwards
      c. Avoid use of deodorants and antiseptics in this area
      d. Wear stockings rather than tights and cotton rather than nylon underclothes
      e. Keep up a high fluid intake, voiding frequently (at least 3 hourly)
   (iv) If after considering (ii) + (iii) there are still problems with recurrent infection, prescribe a 6-month prophylactic course of e.g. nitrofurantoin 100 mg nocte

**Referral**
1. Children. Urinary tract infection in children can cause renal scarring and therefore important to diagnose at an early age. Presentations in infants and those under 3 years (the critical ages) are not classical and hence you must think of UTI in unexplained pyrexia or abdominal pain. A dipslide is useful in this respect. Forty per cent of children with UTI have an underlying anomaly of some sort. Refer after a first proven UTI, regardless of sex
2. Men. Refer because again this may be an anomaly of the urinary tract
3. Women
   (i) Those with gross haematuria may need cystoscopy

(ii)  Women with acute pyelonephritis should have an IVP after the attack

(iii) Recurrent infection. Since this is benign in adults, if there is no evidence of renal disease (proteinuria, hypertension, raised urea and creatinine), can safely refer only those with very frequent and severely disabling attacks. Even then this is more for studies of bladder and urethral function than for an IVP. Consider an ultrasound scan first.

## OBESITY

### Definition
Scientifically speaking the Body mass index is used as the determinate of how fat you are!

$$\text{Body mass index} = \frac{\text{weight (kg)}}{\text{height}^2 \text{ (m}^2)}$$

A value > 25 is overweight, > 30 is obese

e.g. I am 6'2' (1.88 m) and 82 kg:

$$\frac{82}{1.88^2} \qquad \frac{82}{3.53} = 23.2$$

i.e. in the normal range (20–25)

About 5% of the population are at the 30 mark or over

### Management
1. Record height, weight and Body mass index of patient
2. Look at the general health of the patient
   (i)   ? Hypertensive – weight loss will reduce BP
   (ii)  ? Diabetic
   (iii) ? Smoking
   (iv)  ? Psychiatric/family/marital problems – any reason for them being overweight?
   (v)   ? Present medication
   (vi)  ?Cushingoid or hypothyroid
3. Discuss with patient
   (i)   Eating habits – modifying eating behaviour (chewing longer, avoiding snacks, eating only at the table, etc.) is a key part of the management of obesity
   (ii)  Exercise – encourage regular exercise (walking, swimming, jogging)
   (iii) Diet
         a. Usual target is 1000 kcal/day for women and 1500 kcal/day for men
         b. Constituents of the diet should be based on the following principles outlined by the National Advisory Committee on Nutrition Education (NACNE) in their report *Proposals for Nutritional Guidelines for Health Education in Britain*, September, 1983:

Reduce fat content to 30% of total energy intake
Increase ratio of polyunsaturated to saturated fats
Increase fibre intake to 30 g/head/day
Reduce sucrose intake to 20 kg/head/year
Restrict alcohol to less than 4% of calories
Reduce the salt intake
  c. Supply the patient with a diet sheet and recommend
     some books
  d. Some practices have an attached dietitian to go through
     the patient's diet individually
(iv)  Recommend a local self-help group
(v)  Enlist support of the family
4. Follow-up
  (i)  Fortnightly weighing by the nurse
  (ii)  Each patient should keep a diary of intake
  (iii)  With a daily calorie intake of less than 500 kcal of your
     needs, you should lose 0.5 kg/week and this should be the
     aim

**Use of appetite suppressants**
Possibly justified for short-term use in the grossly obese while diet
and behaviour patterns are being modified. Use should be strictly
controlled. Generally best avoided.

# Geriatrics

## PRINCIPLES OF MANAGEMENT OF THE ELDERLY PATIENT

1. Cardinal aim is maintenance of independence, hence concentrate on mobility, stability, continence and intellect
2. Aim to solve specific problems, e.g. How can we help the relatives manage this patient at home?
3. With any problem (falls, constipation, incontinence, etc.) first review the current drug therapy
4. Remember the principles of prescribing for the elderly viz:
   - (i) Keep it under review, especially repeat prescriptions
   - (ii) Ensure drug therapy is necessary, e.g. avoid strong diuretics for minimal ankle oedema
   - (iii) Watch out for adverse reactions and side-effects especially digoxin (take potassium and serum digoxin levels if suspect overdigitalization), pyschotropic drugs, hypnotics and antiparkinsonian agents
   - (iv) Check on compliance
   - (v) Use the minimum number of drugs in appropriate dosage
   - (vi) Use non-steroidal inflammatory drugs (NSAIDs) with discretion in the elderly, due to the risk of gastrointestinal bleeding. Ask about PMH of dyspepsia, peptic ulceration, hiatus hernia, first
   - (vii) Ensure all, including the relatives, understand the rationale for the medication
5. Remember, caring for the elderly is teamwork with the district nurse, health visitor, occupational therapist, social worker, etc.
6. Make sure you know how to organize support services (home helps, meals-on-wheels, etc.) and are aware of local voluntary support services (e.g. offered by Age Concern)
7. Maintain a good liaison with the local hospital geriatricians and the help they can offer (day care, holiday admissions, etc.)
8. Never accept immobility, incontinence or confusion as inevitable or irreversible until the patient has been fully assessed and investigated

9. Look out for some commonly missed treatable causes of disability, i.e.
   (i) Temporal arteritis and polymyalgia rheumatica
   (ii) Hypothyroidism
   (iii) Anaemia, including pernicious anaemia
   (iv) Maturity onset diabetes
10. Pay special attention to vision (cataracts can be removed at any age), deafness (? wax, ? needs a hearing aid) and constipation
11. Remember depression in the elderly can mimic dementia. Antidepressants and even ECT help selected patients

## SCREENING THE ELDERLY

Under the terms of the 1990 Contract, general practitioners are now required to invite (in writing) yearly every patient aged 75 or over to participate in a health promotion consultation and to offer (again in writing) each such person an annual home visit to assess their health care needs. An annual home visit, which can be carried out by a nurse, will fulfil the requirements and will be a regular feature of future general practice. Note that the proportion of the population currently 75+ is about 7% (i.e. 140 patients for an average list of 2000).

For the elderly screening programme to succeed you will need:
1. An up-to-date age–sex register
2. An enthusiastic primary health care team (particularly the practice nurses as they are the most likely members to be undertaking the visits)
3. A good referral system (chiropodists, dietitians, occupational therapists) to cope with the problems uncovered

### The screening protocol

The New Contract lists 6 areas:
1. Sensory functions–assessment of hearing and vision
2. Mobility (? arthritis, ? Parkinson's, ? any recent falls). Consider also here any specific aids required (mobility aids, aids to daily living, home adaptations)
3. Mental condition: ? depressed, ? confused (score by asking specific questions i.e. date, time, address, etc.)
4. Physical condition, including continence. Include here:
   (i) Appearance, ? weight, ? anaemic, ? hypothyroid, ? basal cell carcinoma (common in the elderly), etc.
   (ii) Current medical problems–symptom review including weight, exercise tolerance, dyspnoea and pain
   (iii) Smoking and alcohol
   (iv) Continence–urinary and faecal

    (v) Assessment of cardiovascular system and blood pressure
        (in under 80s)
    (vi) Test of urine for protein and sugar
  5. Social environment
      (i) Accommodation (? warm, ? telephone available)
     (ii) Carers/contact with others
    (iii) Need for help e.g. bath nurses, home help, meals-on-wheels
  6. Use of medicines
     *See* principles of prescribing (p. 28)
The observations made must be noted in the patient's medical
record, although many practices use a special screening card.


## MANAGING A PATIENT WITH A STROKE

### Acute phase
  1. First decision is whether to admit to hospital. Depends on:
      (i) Level of consciousness
     (ii) Age of patient – best to admit if < 65
    (iii) Support at home – the critical factor
  2. Diagnosis. ? Haemorrhage or embolism (with embolism
     consider possibility of recent myocardial infarction or valvular
     disease). In differential diagnosis consider subarachnoid
     haemorrhage, subdural haematoma, cerebral tumour and the
     rarer, but treatable, temporal arteritis and subacute bacterial
     endocarditis. After a stroke check ESR and full blood count (for
     polycythaemia)
  3. Prognosis – poor if reduced level of consciousness, severe
     hemiparesis or conjugate deviation of eyes
  4. Treatment
      (i) In young (< 65) consider rarer differential diagnoses (see
          above) and admit
     (ii) Anticoagulation for those with mitral stenosis and atrial
          fibrillation is a specialist decision
    (iii) No drugs useful in acute stage in the general practice
          setting. Hypertension found, unless BP very high, does not
          need treatment in the acute stage
    (iv) Key treatment is good nursing care with prevention of bed
          sores (? ripple bed), incontinence (? catheter) and
          constipation (? enema). Support family


### Rehabilitation
  1. Spasticity can be helped by baclofen
  2. Dysphasia can be helped by speech therapy
  3. Mobility can be helped by walking aids, physiotherapy as
     available
  4. An occupational therapist will help with feeding problems,
     dressing problems, aids to daily living, etc.

5. Support family and patient. Watch for depression (commonly follows a stroke)
6. Useful leaflets supplied by Chest, Heart and Stroke Association*
7. Consider eligibility for attendance or mobility allowance
8. ? Need for home help or meals-on-wheels

*Note*: GPs may find many of the facilities and therapists available at the local day centre or rehabilitation unit

**Prevention**
1. Control hypertension, particularly in the young and middle-aged
2. TIAs precede 10% of strokes and up to one-third of TIAs progress to a stroke within a year
   (i) Fully assess all those with a TIA (? murmurs, ? atrial fibrillation, ? evidence of myocardial infarction, ? BP, ? carotid bruits plus tests such as FBC, ESR, lipids, blood sugar, etc). Atrial fibrillation in a young person needs referral (after excluding thyrotoxicosis), urgently if associated with heart failure
   (ii) Young patients with a TIA should be referred for consideration of angiography, ? proceed to carotid endarterectomy
   (iii) For prevention use (if no history of peptic ulcer) dispersible or enteric-coated aspirin 300 mg/day (although lower doses may be effective). Warfarin may be more effective than aspirin in certain categories of patient but this will be a specialist decision
3. Detect and prevent risk factors, i.e. obesity, smoking, hyperlipidaemia, diabetes
4. Recognize and treat polycythaemia
5. Anticoagulation with warfarin for
   (i) Those with rheumatic heart disease and atrial fibrillation
   (ii) Those with atrial fibrillation where an embolic episode or a TIA has occurred

**INCONTINENCE**

**Urinary incontinence**

*Assessment:*
1. Test urine for glycosuria and infection
2. Rectal examination for prostatic hypertrophy or faecal impaction
3. In women pelvic examination for atrophic senile vaginitis/prolapse

*Tavistock House North, London WCIH 9JE

4. Review medication – especially strong diuretics, oversedation and anticholinergic drugs causing urinary retention and overflow incontinence
5. Review mental state – incontinence common in confusion and dementia
6. Is patient immobile and unable to get to the toilet?

*Management:*
1. Treat cause
2. Prevent constipation
3. Involve district nurse
4. Use of incontinence pads and pants as appropriate
5. Catheters can be prescribed on an FP10 and changed at home

**Faecal incontinence**
Commonest cause is faecal impaction with overflow incontinence (beware 'diarrhoea' in elderly – often spurious). Rectal prolapse, rectal carcinoma and dementia, other causes
Prevent constipation and ensure regular toileting

**FALLS**

**Causes**
1. Parkinson's disease
2. Drugs – especially oversedation
3. Postural hypotension – including drug-induced
4. Cardiovascular causes, e.g. arrhythmias
5. Transient ischaemic attacks and strokes
6. Metabolic causes: diabetes, anaemia, hypokalaemia, hypothyroidism
7. Fits
8. Drops attacks
9. Disorders of balance, e.g. Ménière's disease
10. Immobility, e.g. due to OA or RA with muscle wasting
11. Confusion

**Assessment**
1. Consider contributory factors, e.g. poor vision, unsafe stairs, etc.
2. Confusion – are the falls a reflection of intellectual impairment?
3. Correctable causes:
   (i) Take a good history: ? fits, ? drop attacks, ? Stokes Adams attacks
   (ii) Examination
      a. Appearance: ? Parkinson's, ? anaemia, ? hypothyroid
      b. Cardiovascular system (CVS): ? arrhythmias, ? erect and supine BP, ? carotid bruits

    c. Central nervous system (CNS): ? weakness, ? ataxia
    d. Joints. Also consider fractured neck of femur as a result
       of a fall
  (iii) Blood test for anaemia, hypothyroidism
  (iv) Urine test for sugar
4. Review medication

## Management

1. Treat correctable causes, e.g. Parkinson's, anaemia, postural
   hypotension (fludrocortisone), arrhythmias (including use of
   pacemakers for heart block), aspirin for TIAs, cervical collar for
   cervical spondylosis, etc.
2. Review how patient is managing at home

## CONFUSION

Distinguish confusion from dementia (Table 4):

**Table 4**

| Acute confusion | Dementia |
| --- | --- |
| Rapid onset | Long history from relatives |
| May be agitated, anxious and hallucinating | Usually placid and calm |
| Performance variable and fluctuating | Performance stable |
| Distant memory affected – often difficult to obtain any history | May retain some distant memory |

## Common causes

1. Change of environment, e.g. moving
2. Drugs especially antiparkinsonians, alcohol, digoxin and
   sedatives
3. Infection, especially respiratory and urinary
4. Cardiac failure/arrhythmias/hypotension/painless myocardial
   infarction
5. Strokes and TIAs
6. Urinary retention
7. Constipation with faecal impaction
8. Pain
9. Dehydration

Less common causes include anaemia, diabetes, uraemia,
hypothermia, hypo- or hyperthyroidism, $B_{12}$ deficiency, head injury.
Social isolation, deafness and blindness contribute

**Assessment**
1. Assess previous history and enquire from relatives
2. Review medication
3. Examination
    (i) General including rectal temperature with low-reading thermometer
    (ii) CVS, remembering painless MI
    (iii) Any signs of chest infection?
    (iv) Abdomen and rectal examination (? urinary retention, faecal impaction)
    (v) CNS – assessment as patient will allow, ? CVA
    (vi) Urine test for sugar
    (vii) If planning management at home FBC, ESR, U and E, T4
4. Record mental state by recording answers to specific questions (day, month, address, year, etc.) – allows for assessment of degree of confusion and useful in monitoring progress

**Management**
1. Treat cause. Occult infection common – trial of an antibiotic may be worthwhile
2. Sedation – most useful are promethazine (Sparine) or thioridazine (Melleril). For nocturnal restlessness try chlormethiazole (Heminevrin)
3. Main decision is whether relatives can cope – if not may need hospital admission and even a section (*see* Psychiatry chapter)


**TERMINAL CARE**

Key areas are:
1. Talking to the patient
    (i) Giving the patient time to express fears
    (ii) Adopting a sympathetic honest approach
    (iii) Allowing the patient to control the pace of the imparting of the information
    (iv) Being sensitive to how much the patient wishes to know
    (v) Visiting regularly and being available
2. Establishing a rapport with the relatives
3. Teamwork
    (i) Involving all members of the primary health care team
    (ii) Working as a team, each adding their own expertise
    (iii) Helping the relatives to cope. In many areas there are nurses specially trained in terminal care. Night nursing services are an essential component
4. Symptom control
    (i) Remembering symptoms other than pain, e.g. cough, dyspnoea, insomnia, constipation
    (ii) Controlling pain

**Principles of pain control**
1. Identify the cause – may be a bedsore or faecal impaction rather than metastases
2. Consider adjuvant therapy with either:
    (i) Drugs (dexamethasone for raised intracranial pressure, antibiotics for infections)
    or
    (ii) Physical measures (drainage of ascites, local injections, nerve blocks, radiotherapy, etc.)
    *Notes*:
        a. NSAIDs are good for bone pain
        b. Do not be afraid to ask the local pain clinic or specialist for help
3. Give analgesia regularly, anticipating the pain. There is no place for prn analgesia
4. Know your analgesics
    (i) For mild pain: paracetamol or aspirin
    (ii) For mild to moderate pain: codeine preparations or co-proxamol
    (iii) For any severe pain: morphine preparations
    *Notes*:
        a. Buprenorphine (Temgesic) is a strong narcotic for moderate to severe pain but often causes vomiting and do not use with morphine (it is an antagonist of it)
        b. Dextromoramide (Palfium) is useful to add to the regular analgesia to control acute exacerbations. Its action only lasts 2 h, hence inappropriate for regular use
        c. A common mistake is waiting too late to start morphine. Start it early
        d. Forms of morphine are:
        Oral tablets – MST, a sustained release preparation useful in home management
        More flexible is 4-hourly oral morphine preparations e.g. Oramorph (Morphine sulphate 2mg/ml) or Oramorph Concentrated (Morphine sulphate 20 mg/ml)
        Diamorphine 4-hourly is the injectable alternative and can be given i.m., s.c. or by subcutaneous infusion. The dose of diamorphine will be about one-third of the dose of morphine in the solution
        e. Titrate the dose of morphine to the pain. Most require 10–30 mg 4-hourly but some need 60 mg or more 4 hourly. Do not be afraid of high doses
        f. With morphine remember
            – To prescribe a prophylactic laxative
            – To write the prescription as a controlled drug (*see* chapter on Prescribing)

5. Be flexible and assess the pain at frequent intervals – daily in the final stages
6. Instruct the relatives how and when to give the analgesia
7. Remember anxiolytics and antidepressants for selected patients, although morphine itself is anxiolytic

*Note:* With teamwork and a committed approach many patients will be able to die at home. Hospital will be needed by some and hospices are increasingly available – for admission of patients and for help and advice

# Psychiatry

## DEPRESSION

### Common presentations of depression in general practice
1. Tiredness – the patient who is 'tired all the time'
2. Insomnia
3. Weight loss and loss of appetite
4. Hypochondriasis – including multiple consultations for vague aches and pains, headaches, giddiness, etc. Delusions of having cancer
5. The patient who complains of feeling depressed
6. The patient who bursts into tears during a consultation
7. The patient with no hope for the future: 'Life's not worth living'
8. Marital problems – as cause or consequence
9. Alcohol problems – as cause or consequence

*Note*: Physical symptoms (tiredness, poor appetite, etc.) as common as psychological symptoms in the initial presentation

### Management of depression in general practice

*Diagnosis*
1. Consider the above presentations
2. Do not be afraid of asking the patient
3. No substitute for personal knowledge of the patient
4. Beware, however, of physical illness masquerading as depression, e.g. the occult carcinoma, hypothyroidism and the early presentations of dementia and Parkinson's disease

*History*
Explore in particular:
1. Recent upheavals and precipitating factors (at work, in the marriage, etc.)

2. Previous history of depression
3. Suicidal intent

*Treatment*
1. Listening and support. May be appropriate to refer to a psychologist, social worker or marriage guidance counsellor
2. Use of antidepressants. Most useful if persistent depression, moderate to severe depression or endogenous features (weight loss, anorexia, early morning wakening, diurnal variation). Least likely to be helpful in mild depression, depression precipitated by a given event and for those with difficulty in coping with life's frustrations
3. Referral, especially for:
   (i) Severe depression, with or without the risk of suicide
   (ii) Recurrent depression or manic depressive illness
   (iii) Those failing to respond to adequate doses of antidepressants for adequate length of time

*Follow-up*
Very important – arrange a follow-up appointment at the outset and reassure patient of your interest and availability

**Use of antidepressants**
Four golden rules:
1. Ensure compliance
   May need to enlist support of relatives, friends and nurses
2. Use adequate dosage
   Often the only difference between GP and psychiatrist is the dosage, e.g. 150 mg of amitriptyline, rather than 75 mg. Aim to build up dose over 10 days in two or three stages. As a rough rule aim for higher-than-average doses in the young (providing drug is tolerated) and half the average in the elderly
3. Continue for an adequate length of time
   Warn patient of 7–10-day delay in onset of action but there should be improvement within 3 weeks. Warn of the possible side-effects. Continue treatment for up to 6 months for maximum benefit and, in any case, for 3 months. Withdraw slowly over 2–3 months
4. Follow up
   Seeing the patient regularly and listening helps problems to be shared and solved

## Choice of antidepressant

**Table 5**

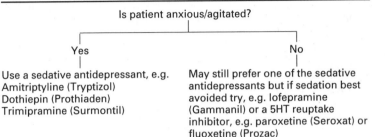

Is patient anxious/agitated?

| Yes | No |
|---|---|
| Use a sedative antidepressant, e.g. Amitriptyline (Tryptizol) Dothiepin (Prothiaden) Trimipramine (Surmontil) | May still prefer one of the sedative antidepressants but if sedation best avoided try, e.g. lofepramine (Gammanil) or a 5HT reuptake inhibitor, e.g. paroxetine (Seroxat) or fluoxetine (Prozac) |

Paroxetine (Seroxat) is also indicated for treatment of depression accompanied by anxiety. The 5HT reuptake inhibitors, such as paroxetine and fluoxetine (Prozac), have comparable efficacy to the tricyclic antidepressants with the advantage of improving sleep disturbance without sedation. As a result they do not impair psychomotor performance. They do not cause the weight gain associated with the tricyclics and are safer in overdose. 5HT reuptake inhibitors are increasingly the first choice for treating depression in general practice

### Side-effects and contraindications of the tricyclics, tetracyclics and related antidepressants

1. Minor anticholinergic side-effects – dry mouth, blurred vision, constipation
2. Cardiac conditions. Cardiotoxic, especially in overdose and use cautiously if cardiac problems. Recent myocardial infarction an absolute contraindication
3. Patients on antihypertensives – antidepressants interfere with some of the older treatments, e.g. methyldopa, but not with the β-blockers
4. Epilepsy – threshold may be lowered and may need to adjust therapy
5. Pregnancy – a contraindication
6. Glaucoma – an attack of glaucoma may be precipitated
7. Prostatic hypertrophy – urinary retention a problem with the tricyclics
8. The elderly – confusional states can be induced and postural hypotension, leading to falls
9. May potentiate the effects of alcohol, phenobarbitone and phenothiazines
10. Do not use within 14 days of the MAOIs and they also interact with levodopa
11. Caution also advised in patients with liver disease, hyperthyroidism and diabetes

## Side-effects of the 5HT reuptake inhibitors
The side-effects of the 5HT reuptake inhibitors tend to be gastrointestinal with nausea having been reported in the first few days of therapy. The incidence of anticholinergic side-effects and postural hypotension is much reduced. There is no cardiotoxicity and no potentiation of the effects of alcohol.

## ANXIETY

### Common presentations of anxiety in general practice
1. Fatigue (but tiredness more a feature of depression)
2. Hyperventilation/breathlessness
3. Palpitations
4. Giddiness/dizziness
5. Paraesthesiae
6. Diarrhoea
7. Dyspepsia
8. Headache
9. Difficulty in sleeping
10. Tremor
11. Lump in the throat, difficulty in swallowing or a dry mouth
12. Psychological symptoms of apprehension, fear of illness, all-pervading worries. Patient may describe himself or herself as 'tense', 'on edge' or 'panicky'

*Note*: Remember thyrotoxicosis!

### Anxiety versus depression
Mixed anxiety and depression common. It has been shown that patients with anxiety plus depression are better treated with an antidepressant than benzodiazepines with their attendant problems of dependence and withdrawal.

In distinguishing the anxiety component from depression consider panic attacks, autonomic symptoms, difficulty getting off to sleep, apprehension and worry as markers of anxiety; and diurnal variation, early morning waking, weight loss, suicidal thoughts and feelings of hopelessness as markers of depression.

### Treatment of anxiety
Possibilities are:
1. Talking to the patient – simple reassurance and support
2. More formal psychotherapy – singly or in groups
3. Relaxation techniques – patient instructed (? use of a tape)
4. Behaviour therapy for phobic anxiety
5. $\beta$-Blockers to control the physical symptoms
6. If patient depressed try a sedative antidepressant, e.g. Prothiaden
7. Short courses of benzodiazepines

*The benzodiazepines*
1. Effective, safe, few side-effects and virtually no drug interactions (apart from alcohol)
2. Warn about driving and operating machinery
3. Can induce a pharmacological dependence in as little as 6 weeks. Dependence may occur in up to one-third of long-term (> 6 months) users
4. Withdraw slowly over 6 weeks with the addition of a $\beta$-blocker to control symptoms
5. Withdrawal symptoms include anxiety, depression, depersonalization, derealization, insomnia, panic attacks, palpitations, sensory disturbances of taste, vision and touch, muscle twitching, paraesthesiae and unsteadiness. Fits and psychosis may be consequent on high dose withdrawal

*Comment:* As yet it is unclear whether use of benzodiazepines is associated with any long-term impairment of mental functioning but, in view of the possibility, it is generally wise to restrict prescribing to short courses of treatment of 2 weeks, i.e. with intermittent rather than continuous treatment. In a selected few patients the quality of life may be so improved by benzodiazepines that the risks of long-term use are outweighed by the clinical benefits – but they should be kept under review.

## MANAGEMENT OF MARITAL PROBLEMS
1. One in three marriages ends in divorce
2. Usually the wife consults but try and involve both
3. May be associated psychiatric problems (depression, alcoholism, etc.) needing help
4. May refer to marriage guidance counsellors – attached to a few practices
5. Support, advise and counsel even if referred

## WHAT TO DO WHEN CONFRONTED WITH A MENTALLY DISTURBED PATIENT REQUIRING ADMISSION TO HOSPITAL
1. Try and defuse the situation. Police may need to be involved if the patient is violent
2. Assess the situation calmly – you will probably know the patient as every practice has its handful of patients intermittently requiring urgent admission
3. You may be able to persuade the patient to accept voluntary admission
4. If the patient refuses but still needs admission you will need a Section. Usually it is not such an emergency that you cannot contact the duty psychiatrist and then both make the medical

**Table 6**    The Mental Health Act 1983

|  | Section 4 | Section 2 |
|---|---|---|
| Broadly equates with or replaces | Section 29 of the 1959 Act | Section 25 of the 1959 Act |
| Main use of the section | Emergency compulsory admission lasting for 72 hours (then converted to a Section 2 or 3.) | Allows admission to hospital for up to 28 days for assessment |
| Medical recommendation | Any doctor, preferably the patient's own GP | Two medical recommendations – one from an 'approved' (i.e. approved under the Act) doctor, usually the psychiatrist |
| Application made by | Patient's nearest relative or an approved social worker | Patient's nearest relative or approved social worker |
| Time intervals | Admission must be within 24 hours of the doctor's examination | The two doctors must have examined the patient within 5 days of each other |

recommendations preferably, but not necessarily, seeing the patient together. The nearest relative (i.e. husband or wife) makes the application or, if not, you must contact an approved social worker. In an emergency situation you can admit under Section 4 (see Table 6), after the application has been made by nearest relative/social worker, but you must then state why using Section 2 (see Table 6) would have involved undesirable delay and why the delay in obtaining the second medical recommendation would have resulted in harm

*Note*: Keep a supply of Section forms in your case and make sure you know how to contact the approved social worker!

## INSOMNIA – REQUEST FOR A HYPNOTIC

Causes of insomnia:
1. External factors – noise, light, heat, etc.
2. An altered lifestyle – shiftwork, international travel, etc.
3. Physical causes – pain, cough, dyspnoea, cramps, etc.
4. Psychiatric causes – depression, anxiety

5. Emotional causes – marital problems, stress at work
6. Drugs, e.g. aminophylline, $\beta$-blockers, alcohol, tea, coffee
7. Unrealistic expectations!

**Management of a patient with insomnia**
1. Look for causes, as above
2. Treat causes whether physical (pain, cough, etc.), psychiatric, emotional or due to drugs
3. Reassure
   (i) Not necessary to have a full night's sleep
   (ii) Sleep is an individual need
   (iii) As you age you need less sleep
4. Advise
   (i) Warm milky drink before going to bed
   (ii) Short walk before bedtime
   (iii) Avoid large meals, exciting books or stimulating TV before going to bed
5. Relaxation techniques may help some
6. Hypnotics. Problems of prescribing a hypnotic are:
   (i) Risk of dependency and rebound insomnia on withdrawal
   (ii) Confusion in the elderly
   (iii) Hangover effect the next morning
   (iv) Effectiveness can lessen or disappear in the first few weeks
   (v) Contraindicated in patients who have sleep apnoea
   Types of benzodiazepine hypnotic are:
   a. Short-acting (6–8 h), e.g. temazepam
   b. Medium-acting (8–12 h), e.g. nitrazepam
   c. Long-acting (over 12 h), e.g. flurazepam (not available at NHS expense)
Cyclopyrrolone (Zimovane) is a non-benzodiazepine hypnotic of use in the short-term treatment of insomnia

## A PATIENT WHO COMPLAINS OF 'TIREDNESS'

In a classic review Valdini (1985) reviewed several reports of patients presenting with fatigue. Of 940 patients the cause was psychological in 57% of cases. Other common causes of tiredness are:
1. Infection, especially glandular fever
2. Cardiovascular causes
3. Endocrine causes: thyroid disorders, diabetes, the menopause
4. Medications
5. Haematological causes, including anaemias
Interestingly, malignancies contributed only 9 out of the 940

**Management**
1. Ask concerning characteristics of the tiredness – severity,

constancy, aggravating factors, etc. Has there been a recent viral illness? What is the current medication?
2. Assess mood. Can a positive diagnosis of anxiety/depression be made?
3. Assess physically – note weight loss, ? anaemic, ? hypothyroid, ? any signs of infection
4. Test the urine for sugar and protein
5. Blood tests as indicated, e.g. full blood count, Paul-Bunnell, T4, TSH

## ALCOHOLISM

1. Presentations of alcoholism/heavy drinking vary in general practice but remember fatigue, anorexia, recurrent nausea and gastritis, insomnia, anxiety, depression and repeated consultations for minor illness. In a wider context remember marital and employment problems
2. Confirmation of the problem
    (i) Interview with the patient
        a. Intake > 4 pints or equivalent/day in a man (one unit of alcohol = glass of wine = single whisky = $1/2$ pint beer) or > 3 pints or equivalent/day in a woman. The RCGP report on alcohol (1986) classified moderate drinkers as men with a weekly consumption of 21–50 units of alcohol and women with a weekly consumption of 16–35 units of alcohol
        b. Patient presents with problems related to, or worsened by, a high alcohol intake
    (ii) High blood alcohol (especially in the morning) or patient smells of alcohol
    (iii) Clinical correlates of alcohol abuse: cirrhosis, tremor, memory loss, etc. Note that only about 10% of alcoholics develop cirrhosis
    (iv) Two important blood tests:
        a. A raised MCV (mean corpuscular volume), the macrocytosis resolving following cessation of alcohol intake
        b. raised γ-glutamyl transpeptidase (γGT) – even if only heavy drinking in the previous few weeks and returns to normal in about 2 months following cessation of alcohol intake
3. Screening. Various screening questionnaires exist, e.g. the CAGE questionnaire or the Michigan alcoholism screening test. Note that fewer than half the alcoholics, and some say only 10% of the heavy drinkers, are known to their general practitioners. It has been estimated that a general practitioner will have about 55 patients on his or her

list whose alcohol consumption poses a high risk (see RCGP, 1986)

**How to manage the heavy drinker/alcoholic in general practice**
1. Recognize the problem
2. Take a full drinking history from the patient with a problem, including reasons for a high alcohol intake
3. Start by encouraging the patient to accept that alcohol is a problem in his or her life
4. Involve the family and friends of the alcoholic – the more support the better the prognosis
5. Advise on
   (i) Benefits of reducing alcohol consumption (on family, finances, work, etc.)
   (ii) Tips to cut down
       a. Do not drink alone
       b. Do not gulp
       c. Do not drink on an empty stomach
6. Help with specific problems, e.g. financial (referral to social services, debt counselling), marital (? marriage guidance counsellor), mental problems (anxiety/depression)
7. Detoxification for the alcoholic can occasionally be carried out at home but only if there is home support, daily supervision and no suicidal risk. Community alcohol teams may help here
8. With each patient set a realistic goal. Controlled drinking is a more realistic initial aim but abstinence should be the aim for those severely addicted and those who do not respond to the controlled approach
9. Maintain motivation by regular follow-up. Monitor progress by patient's and relatives accounts, MCV and γGT. Self-help groups such as Alcoholics Anonymous may help some but the GP's support is essential
10. Get to know the facilities and support available in your area – some areas have community alcohol teams who can be invaluable in the support, supervision and follow-up of those with a drinking problem
11. For a comprehensive review of the management of alcohol-related problems in general practice read the 1986 RCGP Report 24

# ENT

## CAUSES OF EARACHE

1. Trauma
2. Impacted wax
3. Foreign body or furuncle in the ear
4. Otitis externa
5. Otitis media
6. Mastoiditis
7. Neoplasm in the external auditory meatus or middle ear
8. Referred pain from the cervical spine, teeth, sinuses, calculi in the salivary glands, inflammation and malignancy in the nasopharynx, larynx and tonsils and pain from the temporomandibular joint (Costen's syndrome)

## WAX IN THE EAR

1. Before syringing advise patient to use olive oil drops twice a day for 3 days – proprietary preparations can be irritant and are best avoided
2. Use water at body temperature directed upwards and backwards along the canal as shown in Figure 1. Do not aim at the tympanic membrane or you may cause it to rupture or impact the wax against it

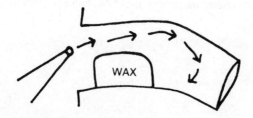

**Fig. 1**

## ACUTE OTITIS MEDIA

Common cause of earache, affecting mainly young children (commonest age about 4–6 years)

**Causes**
Viruses
*Haemophilus influenzae* (under the age of 5 years)
*Streptococcus pneumoniae*
*Streptococcus pyogenes*
*Staphylococcus aureus*
Often follows an upper respiratory tract infection. Blockage of the Eustachian tube may play a major role in the pathogenesis

**Symptoms**
Pain – relieved if the drum perforates
Hearing loss – not often volunteered by children
Discharge – following perforation
Pyrexia, irritability and malaise – in an infant may present solely as a pyrexia or with bouts of screaming

**Signs**
Early: injection of vessels of the handle of the malleus with loss of the light reflex
Middle: tympanic membrane reddens and begins to bulge
Late: perforation and escape of purulent fluid from the middle ear

**Treatment**
1. Pain relief. Regular analgesia important, e.g. paracetamol
2. Antibiotics. Many resolve without but antibiotics may speed resolution and prevent complications. Hence most prescribe for all but the most minor cases. Drug of choice is amoxycillin (more active than penicillin against *Haemophilus* and less gastrointestinal problems than ampicillin). A study by Bain et al (1985) has shown a 2-day high-dose course of amoxycillin (750 mg bd) as effective as the conventional 7–10-day course of amoxycillin 125 mg tds in children age 3–10 years. Jones and Bain (1986) have also shown no difference between a 3-day and a 7-day course of antibiotics
3. Decongestants/antihistamines. The use of nose drops and oral antihistamines or decongestants is of no proven benefit (see Bain, 1983). Best avoided
4. Myringotomy. May relieve persistent pain but now rarely needed

## Follow-up

Standard teaching used to be to follow until hearing returns to normal. This is a heavy workload and it may be sufficient to rely on the mother bringing back the child whose hearing remains impaired. On current evidence I would not recheck after a single episode but if recurrent, persistent, a severe attack or the mother feels the child is deaf weeks after an attack, then a reasonable policy would be to check the drums at 6 weeks with an audiogram at 3 months for those still considered deaf. If more than three attacks of otitis media a year consider referral for adenoidectomy.

## Complications

Mastoiditis

Meningitis and intracranial infection

} Very rare? due to earlier treatment with antibiotics

Chronic suppurative otitis media

? Glue ear – but other factors may be more important, e.g. Eustachian tube dysfunction, allergy and adenoids

## GLUE EAR

Peak incidence at age 3–7 years

## Possible presentations

Deafness

Earache

Poor attention and performance at school

Poor development of language skills

Disobedience at home

*Note:* If the mother thinks her child is deaf she is nearly always right!

## Signs

Tympanic membrane dull, possibly retracted and yellowish or greyish in colour. Occasionally fluid levels seen

Conductive deafness – typically about 30 – 40 dB

## Management

Spontaneous resolution may take months or years but most do resolve eventually, although the child may be deaf in the interim period. Medical treatment with antihistamines and nasal decongestants largely unsuccessful but a 2–4 week trial may help minor cases. Best referred for myringotomy, aspiration of fluid and insertion of grommets, but this approach is increasingly challenged.

Adenoidectomy may also be considered

## OTITIS EXTERNA

### Predisposing causes
Local trauma, e.g. poking the ears, after syringing, etc.
Skin conditions – eczema, psoriasis, seborrhoeic dermatitis
Diabetes mellitus
Foreign body in the ear
Swimming
Certain occupations, e.g. diving, mining, etc.

### Symptoms
Discharge from the ear
Pain and irritation in the ear
Deafness

### Signs
Discharge – may be profuse
Hearing loss – but may have normal hearing
Drum usually normal but must attempt to visualize the drum to
exclude middle-ear disease

### Treatment
1. Aural toilet with cotton wool on a wool carrier (NOT a cotton
   wool bud) or by suction under microscopic control in resistant
   cases
2. Local therapy with ribbon gauze soaked in antibiotic-steroid
   drops (e.g. Locorten-Vioform, Sofradex or Gentisone HC) or by
   drops alone (less efficient). Take care there is no perforation if
   prescribing drops containing aminoglycosides as they are
   ototoxic
3. If chronic, swab for fungi. Otomycosis especially common after
   prolonged therapy with antibiotic drops. For fungal infection try
   Canesten solution or Locorten-Vioform drops
4. Consider the predisposing causes as above. Swimming must
   be avoided for 3 months

### Practical notes
1. Without proper aural toilet, treatment may be disappointing
2. Remember to exclude middle-ear disease as a cause of an
   external otitis
3. Note that sensitivity reactions to the drops may exacerbate
   and prolong the condition (especially neomycin containing
   drops)
4. If otitis persists consider underlying factors, possible missed
   middle-ear disease, fungal infection and sensitivity to the
   drops. May need referral, not least for more aggressive aural
   toilet

## FURUNCLE OF THE AIR

**Cause**
Staphylococci

**Treatment**
Daily ribbon gauze wicks soaked in 10% glycerine in ichthammol,
plus a course of flucloxacillin by mouth
*Note:* Test urine to exclude diabetes if recurrent

## VERTIGO

Many patients present to their GP with 'dizziness' or 'giddiness'.
The first step is to take a proper history and ascertain if the patient
has experienced vertigo – defined as a sense of imbalance
associated with a sensation of movement. The patient feels
themselves or their surroundings rotating, falling or swinging.

**Approach to diagnosis**

Are symptoms

Acute / Chronic/recurrent

| | Acute | Chronic/recurrent |
|---|---|---|
| *History:* | Consider head injury, drugs, alcohol, infection (ask about ENT symptoms and any history of a recent cough, cold, fever or any other viral illness). In the elderly in particular consider a vascular cause. | Ask about deafness, tinnitus, pre-existing ear disease, associated neurological symptoms (visual symptoms, dysarthria, ataxia, etc.). Is there any relation to head position? |
| *Examination:* | Check for nystagmus (a characteristic sign). Ears – tympanic membranes, CNS – briefly! CVS | Check for hearing (? unilateral loss, ? sensorineural loss). Ears – tympanic membranes CNS CVS Check for positional vertigo. In benign paroxysmal positional vertigo a nystagmus and vertigo develops |

(contd)

after a short latent period on moving the patient's head into a critical position and this then fades away after about 20 seconds. There is a decreased response on repeated testing. Nystagmus occurring immediately or persisting on testing (i.e.non-fatiguable) may mean disease of the brain stem or cerebellum, possibly a tumour.

*Common causes*: Labyrinthitis
Vestibular neuronitis
Trauma
Ototoxic drugs, alcohol
Vascular occlusion
Rarely a first attack of Ménière's or multiple sclerosis

Benign paroxysmal positional vertigo. Chronic middle-ear disease. Ménière's disease. Vertebrobasilar ischaemia. Acoustic neuroma. Rarely a posterior fossa tumour or multiple sclerosis

## Practical notes
1. Always take a careful history
2. If recurrent vertigo is associated with unilateral hearing loss refer to exclude an acoustic neuroma
3. In Ménière's there may be severe recurrent attacks of vertigo with vomiting, the associated deafness and tinnitus increasing with the frequency of attacks. However, beware of classifying all recurrent vertigo as Ménière's
4. Most of the common acute causes of vertigo resolve in 3 weeks. If they don't reconsider your diagnosis

## SINUSITIS

### Acute
Usually follows a respiratory infection
Presents with fever, nasal discharge, pain and tenderness in the affected sinuses. May just present as pain in the face, headache or even toothache

Complications (orbital cellulitis, meningitis, cerebral abscess, etc.) are extremely rare

*Treatment*
1. Antibiotics. Augmentin is the antibiotic of choice
2. Analgesia
3. Nasal decongestants for a week (ephedrine or xylometazoline drops)
4. Steam inhalation – instruct the patient to sit over a bowl of boiling water with a towel over their head and Friar's Balsam in the bowl to make the exercise more palatable

## Chronic
X-ray may show mucosal thickening, fluid levels or opacity of the sinus. Medical treatment may help, including oral decongestants. Avoid long-term use of vasoconstrictor nose drops, which can cause a drug-induced rhinitis. Surgery (usually endoscopic) may be necessary. Antral lavage effective but unpopular with patients!

## CAUSES OF A STUFFY NOSE
1. Allergy – hay fever, house-dust mite, animal dusts, etc.
2. Infection – including sinusitis
3. Anatomical obstruction – nasal polyp, foreign body, deviated nasal septum
4. Vasomotor rhinitis
5. Drugs – including methyldopa and long-term use of vasoconstrictor nose drops
6. Tumors – a very rare cause of unilateral obstruction, often with epistaxis and discharge

## EPISTAXIS

### Common causes
1. Trauma (ranging from nose picking to major fractures!)
2. Foreign body
3. Infection (viral or bacterial)
4. Hypertension associated with arteriosclerosis

### Rarer causes
1. Neoplasms of the nose
2. Blood dyscrasias and systemic diseases associated with a haemorrhagic tendency
3. Telangiectasia
4. Use of anticoagulant drugs

**Treatment**
Three aims: assess the blood loss, identify the cause and stop the bleeding!

*The younger patient*
In children and young adults bleeding is usually from the anterior part of the nasal septum from veins at the edge of Little's area.
1. Advice. Firm, sustained pressure by pinching the nostrils between finger and thumb for 10 min by the clock with the patient breathing through the mouth. Pressure must be continuous. A sponge or towel soaked in cold water, or an ice-pack over the bridge of the nose reduces blood flow
2. If bleeding does not stop, try again. If bleeding continues you will need to pack the nose with ribbon gauze impregnated with BIPP, using a Thudichum's speculum and nasal forceps. A technique worth learning

*The middle-aged and elderly*
Here bleeding may well be arterial and can be profuse, persistent and even life-threatening. Note the BP and check how much blood has been lost – it may be a significant quantity. Probably best packed in hospital if severe or the simple advice regimen fails to halt the bleeding. May even need arterial ligation

**Recurrent epistaxes**
Quite common in children and young adults. After excluding an underlying cause (including a blood count), the vessels can be cauterized, under local anaesthesia, by electric cautery, trichloroacetic acid or a silver nitrate stick.

## SORE THROAT

**Common causes**
1. Viruses (more than half of acute sore throats are of viral origin. Glandular fever, caused by the Epstein-Barr virus, is a less common cause of a sore throat)
2. Bacteria – streptococci, pneumococci, staphylococci, *Haemophilus influenzae*
3. Smoking and other local irritants (alcohol, fumes, foreign bodies, overuse of medications for the throat, gastric reflux $\pm$ hiatus hernia)

**Rarer causes**
1. Candidiasis
2. Aphthous ulceration

3. Tumors of the oropharynx, base of the tongue and
   hypopharynx
4. Rare infections, e.g. Vincent's angina, tuberculosis, syphilis,
   AIDS and, of course, diphtheria
5. Blood dyscrasias, including agranulocytosis. Leukaemia can
   present as a persistent throat ulceration

**History**
The length and severity of the symptoms. Any associated
symptoms

**Examination**
Examine the throat and feel the neck for lymphadenopathy

**Investigations**
Throat swabs are largely a waste of time. Only used for suspected
rare causes. If sore throat fails to resolve in 10 days consider
glandular fever and order a full blood count and a Paul-
Bunnell/Monospot test. If both these are normal and the sore throat
is still persisting consider some of the rarer causes and the possible
need for referral.

**Treatment**
By far the vast majority of sore throats will be infective, mainly of
viral origin, and there are two options:
1. Simple advice: soluble aspirin gargles and throat lozenges for a
   few days to relieve the soreness
2. Treat with penicillin (as the commonest bacterial cause is
   streptococci). If allergic to penicillin try erythromycin. Do not
   use ampicillin – may produce a rash if the patient has
   glandular fever. Prescribe a 7 – 10-day course. If a purulent
   tonsillits, consider giving the initial dose by intramuscular
   injection
Patient expectation of a prescription for an antibiotic is high. You
must decide yourself what your policy will be. Whereas for a
purulent sore throat in a febrile child an antibiotic might seem
justified, for a minor sore throat in an adult a prescription might not
be the appropriate response. There is little clinical evidence to
support a prescription for penicillin for an afebrile patient with a
simple sore throat. Even for a true streptococcal sore throat the
prescription of an antibiotic has been shown to shorten the illness
by only 12 – 48 h.

**Penicillin allergy**
True overall incidence of allergic reactions lies between 1 and 10%.
Anaphylactic shock very rare (incidence less than 0.02% and even
then largely confined to injections of penicillin)

### Referral
1. Quinsy (a peritonsillar abscess). Characterized by acute severe pain, trismus and inability to swallow. There is marked swelling and pyrexia
2. Unilateral tonsillar enlargement – there may be an underlying pathology
3. Repeated tonsillitis (see below)
4. The unresolving sore throat with no apparent cause

*Note*: Rheumatic fever and glomerulonephritis as complications of a streptococcal sore throat are now extremely rare

## GLANDULAR FEVER
Occurs mainly in the 15–25-year-old age group

### Common symptoms
Fever and malaise
Sore throat unresponsive to antibiotics and persisting longer than 7 days
Swollen neck glands.

### Signs
Exudate or pseudomembrane over the enlarged swollen tonsils
Palatal petechiae
Lymphadenopathy – may be gross cervical lymphadenopathy and palpable occipital nodes
Rash – especially if given ampicillin
Splenomegaly (about 50%)

### Investigations
Full blood count shows atypical lymphocytes

*Antibodies*
The heterophile antibody is detected by the Paul-Bunnell/Monospot test which is positive in about 80% of cases. Antibody production can be slow and may need to repeat test in 2 weeks to confirm the diagnosis. Can remain positive for many months. There are more sensitive methods to detect antibodies to the Epstein-Barr virus, but not in routine use.
Liver function tests abnormal in over 80% of cases but less than 10% of patients are jaundiced.

### Differential diagnosis
Includes cytomegalovirus and toxoplasmosis

### Complications
Usually none but can be many! Reasonably common are severe

pharyngeal swelling (for which steroids may be prescribed) and a prolonged lethargy and depression lasting for months after the acute phase

**Treatment**
Symptomatic – steroids have been tried for some of the complications

## INDICATIONS FOR TONSILLECTOMY

1. Recurrent attacks of tonsillitis, e.g. five attacks a year for 2 years. More important is the time taken off school/work
2. A quinsy
3. Tonsillar hypertrophy sufficient to cause respiratory obstruction and right-sided heart failure. In general, enlargement of the tonsils is not an indication for operation but a small group of children have grossly hypertrophied tonsils causing sleep apnoea and cor pulmonale. Since this can be fatal, operation is essential in this group
4. Unilateral tonsillar enlargement – since there may be an underlying pathology

Recurrent tonsillitis with recurrent otitis media is usually dealt with by both tonsillectomy and adenoidectomy. The place of tonsillectomy in patients with a carditis or a nephritis is disputed.

# Ophthalmology

**Table 7**   Causes of a red eye

|  | Conjunctivitis | Acute iritis | Acute glaucoma | Keratitis |
|---|---|---|---|---|
| Pain | Gritty | + | Severe | Variable |
| Vision | Normal | Blurred | Reduced | Variable |
| Discharge | + | Watery | None or slight | Watery + discharge |
| Site of redness | Peripheral | Circumcorneal | Diffuse | Diffuse or circumcorneal |
| Pupil size | Normal | Small | Dilated oval | Normal |
| Pupil response to light | Normal | Poor | Fixed | Normal |
| Cornea | Clear | Clear + deposits |  |  |

## CONJUNCTIVITIS

1. Common, bilateral
2. Infective with discharge/sticky eyes. Allergic may present just as watering plus itching
3. Bacterial conjunctivitis treated by frequent (initially hourly) chloramphenicol eye drops plus ointment at night for 4–5 days until cleared. Continue for 48 h after eye looks normal
4. Opticrom treatment of choice for allergic conjunctivitis

## ACUTE IRITIS

1. Blurred vision with photophobia and small pupil

2. Refer at once for treatment with steroid and atropine eye drops to a consultant. A threat to sight

## ACUTE GLAUCOMA

1. Pain severe, often with vomiting
2. Eye hard and tender. Vision grossly reduced
3. May be preceded by subacute attacks with haloes around lights
4. Refer immediately (sight can be lost in hours) giving immediate 4% pilocarpine eye drops every few minutes to try and constrict the pupil while awaiting the ophthalmologist

## KERATITIS

Inflammation of the cornea due to infection or trauma
Herpes simplex virus an infective cause, the corneal ulcer being demonstrated with fluorescein. DO NOT USE STEROIDS. Refer

## PRACTICAL POINTS

1. Beware the unilateral red eye and the painful red eye
2. Adopt a methodical approach to examination of the eye (visual acuity, visual fields, eye movements, lids, cornea, pupil, intraocular pressure, ophthalmoscopy, fluorescein staining). Fluorescein staining important but make sure first that patient not wearing contact lenses (lenses will take up the stain)!
3. Steroid-containing eye drops can cause blindness in cases of Herpes simplex keratitis and can raise intraocular pressure. Never use in the undiagnosed red eye and never until fluorescein has shown the corneal epithelium to be intact. Best used under consultant supervision

## TREATMENT OF SOME COMMON EYE PROBLEMS IN GENERAL PRACTICE

### Style

1. Usually discharges spontaneously
2. Instil Chloromycetin drops to sac and ointment to the lid margins
3. If pointing remove the lash to allow drainage
4. With recurrent styes test for diabetes and add a course of flucloxacillin

### Blepharitis (inflammation of the lid margins)

1. Try hygiene of the lids, removing scales with a bud soaked in saline and massaging Chloromycetin ointment into the lids twice a day for 3 weeks

2. Treat associated dandruff
3. If resistant try Chloromycetin hydrocortisone ointment (not if a history of, or there is a suspected associated, herpes keratitis)

### Chalazion (meibomian cyst)
1. If infected try Chloromycetin ointment. Some resolve spontaneously
2. If not resolving or uninfected, surgical curettage needed

### Subconjunctival haemorrhage
1. None. Rarely associated with hypertension and, if recurrent, consider blood dyscrasias
2. If associated with trauma refer (? penetrating foreign body, etc.)

### Dry eyes
1. Common, especially in the elderly. May be associated with systemic disorders, e.g. rheumatoid arthritis
2. After full ophthalmological assessment treatment is artificial tears, e.g. Liquifilm

## TRAUMA TO THE EYE

### Chemical burns
Alkalis the worst. After immediate copious irrigation with water, refer to hospital as an emergency

### Blows to the eye
Refer. A hyphaema is a sign of serious injury and these must certainly be referred. Shotgun pellets and squash balls are notorious

### Foreign body in the eye
1. Most important is the history. If any history of hammering, chiselling, banging or grinding, i.e. a flying particle with possible penetrating injury of the eye, refer at once. Also refer if any suggestion of a metallic foreign body irrespective of the above
2. Learn the technique of removing a foreign body from the eye

## CAUSES OF A SUDDEN LOSS OF VISION (OTHER THAN CAUSES OF ACUTE RED EYE)
1. Retinal detachment
2. Central retinal vein occlusion
3. Central retinal artery occlusion – remember emboli from various sources and temporal arteritis
4. Trauma/chemical toxins

5. Vitreous haemorrhage – hypertension and diabetes are causes
6. A cerebrovascular accident
7. Migraine
8. Optic neuritis

## PRINCIPAL CAUSES OF CHRONIC VISUAL LOSS

1. Cataract
2. Glaucoma
3. Senile macular degeneration
4. Diabetes mellitus

## SCREENING FOR GLAUCOMA

1. Affects 1% of the population over 40 years
2. Early diagnosis and treatment can prevent blindness
3. Screening is possible in general practice, using a tonometer
4. Since there is a strong familial element, particularly important to screen first-degree relatives

## FLOATERS AND FLASHES

1. Key to the urgency of referral is the length of the history
2. Acute onset of 'floaters', 'flashes' or 'lights', floaters associated with a change in vision or appearing in a diseased eye all merit serious consideration. Showers of flashing lights may indicate a retinal tear or detachment, preceding the visual loss and requiring immediate urgent referral
3. Acute onset of floaters can also be due to vitreous haemorrhage
4. Flickering lights can be a feature of migraine
5. Simple vitreous floaters are annoying to patients, may last a long time but are of no significance

## WHAT TO REFER IN OPHTHALMOLOGY – SOME IMPORTANT REFERRALS

1. Herpes zoster ophthalmicus – risk of eye complications
2. Herpes simplex keratitis
3. Red eye if in doubt of diagnosis, especially the unilateral or painful red eye
4. Acute iritis: refer immediately
5. Acute glaucoma: refer immediately
6. Trauma – except minor foreign bodies easily removed
7. Chronic glaucoma – suspect if family history, history of haloes around lights, intermittent blurring of vision, cupping of optic disc, visual field loss

8. Cataracts, if the decreased visual acuity is significantly interfering with patient's life, but remember problems postcataract extraction and select patients carefully

9. Diabetics with a retinopathy need expert assessment and follow-up

10. Most causes of acute visual loss. Beware of missing retinal detachment and temporal arteritis. Note that with some vascular occlusions, sight can be saved in hours – important to refer urgently

11. Squint. Refer constant squints as early as possible in the first weeks of life. Retinoblastoma can present as squint. Inconstant squints need referral if persisting after 6 months. Early treatment of squint essential

12. A mixed bag of less common causes including proptosis, recurrent episcleritis, ectropion and entropion (both for plastic surgery), orbital cellulitis. Nasolacrimal duct obstruction should not generally be referred before 9 months as the ducts may not canalize naturally before this age

# Dermatology

## DIFFERENTIAL DIAGNOSIS OF A SCALY RASH

Psoriasis
Eczema
Tinea
Lichen planus
Pityriasis rosea
Lupus erythematosus

## PRURITUS

Causes of generalized pruritus
  1. Systemic
  – Allergic reactions, e.g. to drugs
  – Diabetes mellitus
  – Hypothyroidism or thyrotoxicosis
  – Malignancies
  – Hodgkin's disease
  – Some myeloproliferative disorders
  – Chronic renal failure
  – Iron deficiency
  – Cholestasis
  2. Psychological
  3. Skin disorders
  – Eczema
  – Lichen planus
  – Dermatitis herpetiformis
  – Urticaria
  – Infestations, e.g. scabies
  4. Senile pruritus. Due to ischaemic and atrophic changes

## PSORIASIS

2% of UK population affected
Red plaques with silvery scales, commonly on elbows and knees.

Can affect scalp and nails and may be associated with an arthropathy.

**Management**
1. Explanation to patient:
   Not contagious
   Does not scar
   Does not affect organs other than skin
2. Topical therapy
   (i) Topical steroids
       a. Useful for groin, axilla, breasts, hands and feet
       b. Potent steroids, e.g. Betnovate, /Dermovate should not
          be used > 3 weeks. They are used to induce short-term
          remission
       c. Polythene occlusion will increase the potency when
          used on hands and feet
       d. Problems of topical steroids include rebound
          exacerbation, side-effects (see below) and danger of
          excess use as patient finds them acceptable
   (ii) Dithranol – for stable plaque psoriasis
       a. Not for face or flexures
       b. 'Short contact therapy' with Dithrocream effective for
          plaque psoriasis. Dithrocream applied for 30 min per
          day, then washed off – start with 0.1% Dithrocream and
          increase weekly, according to response, from 0.1% to
          0.25% to 0.5% to 1% but note some people are very
          sensitive and cannot tolerate dithranol
          4–6 weeks treatment is usually sufficient
   (iii) Tar preparations
       a. Daily applications of crude coal tar in zinc paste may be
          used, but messy
       b. Tar baths used in addition, e.g. using Polytar Emollient
       c. Newer tar preparations many find less effective
   (iv) Calcipotriol (Dovonex):
       – A vitamin D analogue highly acceptable to patients and
         now often used as first-line topical treatment of mild to
         moderate plaque psoriasis
       – Contraindicated in those with disorders of calcium
         metabolism and if patient is using > 80 g/week it is
         probably wise to check the serum calcium occasionally
         (e.g. every 2 months)
       – Not for use on the face
3. Other treatments. Hospital-based and include PUVA
   (methoxy psoralen plus u.v. light), methotrexate and etretinate
   therapy
4. For the scaly scalp try Ung Cocois Co rubbed in every night for
   a few days and washed off every morning – this reduces the

scales and can be followed by 2 weeks use of Betnovate Scalp Application

## ECZEMA

### Clinical types
1. Exogenous – caused by irritants (detergents, oils, etc.) or sensitivity (e.g. to nickel). In hand eczema especially consider exogenous factors
2. Atopic – associated with a family history of atopy (asthma, hay fever, etc.). Commonly starts on face in infancy, localizing to flexures as child gets older
3. Seborrhoeic – in infant presents as cradle cap, nappy rash or more generalized. In adult affects scalp (dandruff), face, trunk and intertriginous areas
4. Varicose eczema
5. Discoid – an eruption of vesicles and exudation on extensor surfaces
6. Pompholyx – collections of large blisters on hands and feet. Distinguish from exogenous eczema
7. Asteatotic eczema – a dry eczema in the elderly

### Management of eczema

*Acute*
1. Is there an exogenous factor?
2. Is it infected – if so prescribe antibiotics
3. If acutely inflamed and weeping eczema involving hands and feet, including pompholyx, try 1:8000 potassium permanganate soaks for 15 min three times a day
4. Use steroid lotions and creams when acute phase is settling

*Chronic*
1. Classify into one of the clinical types
2. Explanation to patient
3. Look for irritants or aggravating factors
4. General measures, e.g. avoidance of soap and use of emulsifying ointment as soap substitute. For dry skin Oilatum Emollient in bath effective, including for infants
5. Systemic therapy
    (i) Antibiotics for infected, crusting eczema. Also try for 'resistant' eczema
    (ii) Antihistamines – especially for children (e.g. Vallergan)
    (iii) Oral steroids – very rarely
6. Topical corticosteroids
    (i) For atopic and seborrhoeic – mild
    (ii) Discoid and pompholyx – may need potent

(iii) When treating intertriginous areas (axillae, submammary and groins) avoid ointments and potent steroids as absorption will be high. Infection common in these sites and it may be wise to use combined topical corticosteroid plus antifungal/antibiotic, e.g. Daktacort

**Notes on the use of topical corticosteroids**
1. Potency – see table in MIMS. A potency ladder would be:
   Hydrocortisone
   Eumovate
   Betnovate          Increasing potency
   Dermovate
2. Ointments more effective than creams but greasy and hence less acceptable. Ointments preferred for areas of dry and scaly skin, whereas creams better for moist or weeping lesions
3. Contraindications include acne, rosacea, infections, perioral dermatitis and immediately surrounding a leg ulcer
4. Side-effects
   (i) Cutaneous atrophy – can occur after only a month of potent steroid, especially on face and flexures, and because of polythene occlusion. Telangiectasia, striae, purpura and poor wound healing result
   (ii) Perioral dermatitis of face. Can also aggravate acne and rosacea
   (iii) Adrenal suppression – 50 g Dermovate/week for 3 weeks can cause it in an adult, possibly with less, and in children as little as 15 g/week
   (iv) Topical steroids near the eye can precipitate glaucoma
   (v) Infection – skin infection exacerbated, tinea infections spread and assume atypical forms
   (vi) Can get an allergic contact dermatitis to the steroid preparation itself
5. Combination preparations available, e.g. steroid and antibiotic (e.g. Fucidin H)
6. About 30 g of cream or ointment covers an adult's skin once
7. Rules concerning use are:
   (i) Only use hydrocortisone on face
   (ii) If using potent steroids (not hydrocortisone), limit to 50 g/week in an adult and 15 g/week in a child
   (iii) With children use less potent preparations
   (iv) Be wary using in flexures or with polythene occlusion – penetration increased in both instances
   (v) Instruct patient fully and review rather than repeat prescription if a potent steroid being used

## CRADLE CAP

Clears in a few months, helped by rubbing olive oil into scalp. If severe try low-dose sulphur and salicylic acid cream applied at night and shampooed out the next morning

## DANDRUFF

First try shampooing with simpler shampoos, e.g. Cetavlon. Polytar shampoo, also used in psoriasis, worth a try. If dandruff severe, choice is between 2% salicylic acid and 2% sulphur cream three times a week (applied nightly and shampooed out next morning) or Betnovate Scalp Application starting with night and morning applications

## MANAGEMENT OF FIVE COMMON SKIN DISORDERS IN GENERAL PRACTICE

1. Urticaria
    (i) Acute with angio-oedema: s.c. adrenaline (0.5 ml of 1 in 1000)
       +200 mg i.v. hydrocortisone
       +10 mg i.v. chlorpheniramine (Piriton)
       If laryngeal obstruction may need a tracheotomy
   (ii) Prolonged attacks may need a short course of oral steroids
   (iii) For simple or chronic urticaria:
       a. Antihistamines, e.g. terfenadine (Triludan)
       b. Search for trigger factors
          Avoid aspirin and codeine
          Avoid foods containing tartrazine, benzoates and salicylates. E numbers to avoid include E102 (tartrazine), E210 (benzoic acid), E104, E110, E210–E219
2. Acne vulgaris
    (i) Topical therapy – three options for use in mild acne
       a. Benzoyl peroxide preparations, starting with 5% once daily for a few hours, then if response poor, increasing after 2 weeks to twice daily, then to 10%. Mild erythema and peeling to be expected but some people unduly sensitive, and cannot tolerate. Reassess in 3 months
       b. Tretinoin (Retin-A) can be more effective if comedones present – can also be used with benzoyl peroxide (one in morning, one in evening). Warn of sensitivity to sunlight
       c. Topical antibiotics, e.g. 1% clindamycin lotion (Dalacin T), erythromycin solution (Stiemycin) or tetracycline solution (Topicycline). Remember to stop Dalacin T if diarrhoea (rare danger of pseudomembranous colitis)

(ii) Systemic therapy – for use in moderate acne

    a. Antibiotics (can be used with topicals), e.g. oxytetracycline or erythromycin 500 mg bd for 3 months then 250 mg bd for 3–6 months (higher dose or longer dose as required). Oxytetracycline not to children, in pregnancy or with milk. Minocycline 50 mg bd an expensive alternative

    b. Dianette – also a contraceptive. Only for refractory acne in women unresponsive to the above. Monitor use (see literature)

(iii) Isotretinoin (Roaccutane) For hospital use only for patients with severe acne

(iv) Advice

    a. On treatment – stress long course

    b. No need for a diet

    c. Wash areas regularly at least twice a day

3. Ringworm (tinea)

  (i) Topical therapy – Imidazoles, e.g. miconazole (Daktarin) for at least 3 weeks. Acute tinea pedis best treated initially with potassium permanganate (1:8000) soaks 10–15 min four to six times a day

  (ii) Systemic therapy – griseofulvin 500 mg – 1 g daily for scalp infections, nail infections (fingernails 6 months, toenails longer) or more severe body infections. Taken with food – warn patient of headache and nausea. Dose for children 10 mg/kg body weight. Contraindicated in liver disease, may cause drowsiness and may reduce the effect of warfarin and the oral contraceptive. Terbinafine (Lamisil) a new alternative to griseofulvin

Note: Skin scrapings examined with a microscope on a slide in 10% potassium hydroxide will demonstrate hyphae

4. Scabies

Treat all the family

Lorexane applied to whole body except head and neck and washed off after 24 h, repeating after 4 days as required

5. Verrucae

Salactol paint applied every night for 6–12 weeks

Prior to application rub with pumice stone or manicure emery paper. Cryocautery an alternative if very large

## PITYRIASIS ROSEA

A skin rash commonly seen in general practice. Starts with solitary herald patch. Within 7–10 days widespread rash, largely on trunk of oval lesions with a collar of scale at their edge and following the cleavage lines. Resolves with no sequelae in 2–3 months

# Paediatrics

The most common presentations in general practice are:
1. Respiratory problems – coughs, asthma and croup
2. ENT problems – otitis media, tonsillitis and epistaxis
3. Skin problems – infantile eczema, nappy rash, verrucae, threadworms and, in older children, acne
4. Infectious illness – mumps, chickenpox, rubella, measles, other viral illnesses
5. Accidents and injuries – head injuries, lacerations, bruises, ingestions, etc.
6. Diarrhoea and vomiting
7. Conjunctivitis
8. Abdominal pain
9. Behaviour problems – crying, feeding problems, encopresis and enuresis
10. Preventative work – immunization and developmental assessment

## FOURTEEN DIAGNOSES NOT TO MISS IN CHILDREN/INFANTS

1. Meningitis – in any sick or febrile child this is *the* diagnosis to exclude
2. Intussusception – remember in the screaming child
3. Epiglottitis – distinguish from croup
4. Hernia – infants with an inguinal hernia need immediate referral for surgery
5. Dehydration after diarrhoea and/or vomiting – do not underestimate
6. Appendicitis – uncommon in children but may rapidly progress to perforation
7. Diabetes mellitus
8. Asthma – underdiagnosed. Consider especially the child with a recurrent cough
9. Torsion of the testis – more often in the older child/adolescent. Refer at once – minutes matter
10. Perthes' disease – beware the child with a limp.

11. Urinary tract infection – important not to miss. Pyrexia with no obvious cause merits a urine culture. One proven UTI means referral for IVP/scan, etc. Renal damage can occur at an early age and may be preventable – *see* Medical chapter
12. Non-accidental injury – the GP has a key role
13. Failure to thrive – all GPs should have percentile charts of height and weight
14. Developmental problems, especially
    (i) Congenital dislocation of the hip – vital it is detected early
    (ii) Squint – *see* Ophthalmology chapter
    (iii) Undescended testes
    (iv) Hearing defects
    (v) Scoliosis

## THE CHILD WITH CROUP

Common cause of a night visit. Distinguish from the two other causes of stridor: epiglottitis and an inhaled foreign body (see Table 8)

*Notes:-*
1. NEVER examine the throat of a child with stridor – if epiglottitis, may precipitate complete airways obstruction

**Table 8**

|  | Croup | Epiglottitis |
|---|---|---|
| Usual age of child | 6 months–3 years | 2–7 years |
| Cause | Parainfluenza virus | *Haemophilus influenzae* |
| Fever | Often none or mild | > 38°C |
| Look of child | May not look too ill Sometimes can eat/drink | Looks ill, toxic, tachycardia |
| Length of illness | Often preceded by a prodromal coryzal illness | Rapid course – progressing in hours |
| Stridor | Loud | Muffled – quieter than croup |
| Sore throat | – | + |
| Dysphagia, drooling saliva | – | + |
| Posture |  | Child prefers sitting upright |

Unfortunately, Table 8 is only a guide and not always 100% reliable

2. Acute stridor of sudden onset with no illness suggests an inhaled foreign body
3. Assess the degree of respiratory obstruction. Signs of severity are:
    (i)   Cyanosis – an emergency
    (ii)  Generalized restlessness or drowsiness
    (iii) Tachycardia
    (iv)  Intercostal recession and accessory muscle respiration
    (v)   Continuous stridor
4. Refer urgently a child with signs of obstruction – epiglottitis is one instance where the GP should accompany the child to Casualty. An inhaled foreign body may cause immediate obstruction necessitating an emergency tracheostomy – make sure you know how to do one

**Treatment**
1. Treatment of croup is steam inhalation, sitting the child in a bathroom full of steam or boiling a kettle in the bedroom. Instruct the parents when to call for a revisit if the child's condition deteriorates – croup itself can cause sufficient respiratory obstruction to merit referral
2. Admit all cases where there is any suspicion of epiglottitis as an emergency
3. Telephone advice for 'croup' is fraught with danger – visit all children with stridor

## THE CHILD WITH ENURESIS

Enuresis is failure to voluntarily control micturition. Can be diurnal or nocturnal. 10% of 5-year-olds wet their beds. Treatment is justified after the age of 4 years

**History**
1. Primary or secondary? Secondary may be emotional or organic
2. Are there other symptoms, e.g. dysuria, abdominal pain?
3. Family history?
4. Is the child developing normally, both mentally and physically?
5. Any stresses in the family?
6. Parents' expectations? Are they referring the child too early (i.e. before 4 years)?

**Examination**
1. Examine the back and lower limbs for anatomical anomalies or lesions of the lower spinal cord
2. Palpate the abdomen for kidneys and bladder and examine the external genitalia of boys

**Tests**
1. Test the urine for protein and sugar
2. Send the urine to be cultured for bacteriuria

**Management**
With no anomalies, neuropathic bladder or UTI, the management is:
1. Advice, e.g. lifting the child before going to sleep
2. Star charts, rewarding the child for dry nights and reviewing the chart to encourage success
3. Enuresis alarms cure 80% in 6 months and are the treatment of choice. Relapse responds to restarting the alarm. Best for the 6+ age group, as a little frightening at 5 years old. Health visitors ideally suited to educating parents and following up children with enuresis
4. Desmospray is now the first-choice drug treatment for nocturnal enuresis especially for the 7+ age group. There is, however, a significant relapse rate. An occasional child will still respond better to imipramine (Tofranil) – dose is 25 mg nocte at age 6–7 and 25–50 mg nocte in the 8–11 year old. Imipramine has the disadvantages of potentially serious side-effects (e.g. agranulocytosis) and it may be fatal in overdose

**Notes**
1. GPs can manage most cases of enuresis in conjunction with the health visitor
2. Enuresis may be just one of a range of behavioural problems
3. Remember to refer and follow up children with UTIs

### THE CHILD WITH A FEBRILE CONVULSION

Affects 3–4% of children, chiefly between the ages of 1–4$\frac{1}{2}$ years. Often a family history

**Management**
1. Ensure a clear airway and that the child is lying in the left lateral position
2. Stop the convulsion with parenteral diazepam. In young children rectal diazepam is the most convenient, using Stesolid rectal tubes (dose is 5 mg for 1–3 years and 10 mg for over 3 years). Intravenous route rarely practical – dose is 0.1 – 0.25 mg/kg body weight
3. Lower the temperature by discarding clothes, tepid sponging and paracetamol elixir
4. Determine the cause – often an otitis media or a tonsillitis. Main task is to exclude a meningitis and also remember UTI. Wisest to admit a child after its first febrile convulsion but with febrile

convulsions in subsequent illnesses admission depends on the diagnosis. Can educate parents in the use of Stesolid but obviously the GP still needs to be called to determine the diagnosis

**Prophylaxis**
1. Simple febrile convulsions (< 15 minutes, no focal features, in normally developing children aged 1–5 years) are not associated with intellectual retardation or long-term neurological disorder. The risk of later epilepsy is only about 1%. Complex convulsions (> 15  minutes, focal signs, onset before 1 year old) may be associated with later temporal lobe epilepsy
2. Prophylaxis with anticonvulsants should be considered in those with recurrent or complex/atypical convulsions. Best to decide by discussion of each child with the paediatrician

## THE INFANT WITH 'DIARRHOEA AND VOMITING'

**Causes**
These include:
1. Tonsillitis and otitis media
2. Intussusception
3. Meningitis – may be atypical in infants
4. Pneumonia
5. Urinary tract infection
6. Gastroenteritis

Parents' history may not be exact and vomiting may be a non-specific symptom of an ill baby. Hence vital to examine fully every infant with 'diarrhoea and/or vomiting'

**Management**
If serious disease suspected, refer
1. If a simple gastroenteritis, assess dehydration from the length of the history, the frequency of the diarrhoea and vomiting, and the signs
2. Signs of dehydration (occur when baby is > 5% dehydrated)
   (i) Loss of skin elasticity – doughy skin
   (ii) Weight loss
   (iii) Oliguria, i.e. fewer wet nappies
   (iv) Tachycardia and tachypnoea
   (v) Sunken eyes with no tears
   (vi) Sunken fontanelle
   (vii) Dry mouth
   (viii) Irritability or lethargy

IF THERE ARE SIGNS OF DEHYDRATION, ADMIT
Management of simple gastroenteritis in infants is:

(i) Advice – no milk or solid food for 24–48 h
(ii) Clear fluids to be given – the ideal is a glucose electrolyte solution, e.g. Dioralyte sachets. Advise small sips often – intake should be about 1–1$1/2$ times the usual feed volume
(iii) Review the next day, within 24 h. Tell the parents to contact you earlier if the infant refuses all fluid, the vomiting increases, the infant's condition deteriorates or other complications develop
(iv) On review, if infant still vomiting or signs of dehydration evident, admit. If child improving, continue Dioralyte and then begin, as symptoms settle, to regrade though $1/4$ strength to $1/2$ strength and finally to full strength feeds in 12–24-h steps according to progress
(v) Recurrence of diarrhoea occasionally due to lactose intolerance – if so try a soya milk, e.g. Wysoy, for a month
(vi) Social circumstances and parental attitudes obviously important in determining management
(vii) A written advice sheet is helpful
(viii) If breastfed the baby can continue – giving little and often, supplemented with Dioralyte

## DIARRHOEA AND VOMITING IN OLDER CHILDREN

Much more likely to be just a simple gastroenteritis rather than a manifestation of other illness, but remember appendicitis

## THE INFANT WITH A NAPPY RASH

Simple nappy rash responds to frequent nappy changes, leaving nappies off for part of the day, and zinc and castor oil cream as a barrier. If severe or resistant, it may mean infection with *Candida albicans* – try Nystaform – HC or Timodine

## THE CHILD WITH A COUGH

Commonly due to simple respiratory tract infections but if persistent think of:
1. Pertussis – *see* chapter on Infectious diseases
2. Asthma
3. Inhaled foreign body
4. Chronic respiratory infection secondary to a postnasal drip from infected sinuses or adenoids
5. Anatomical anomalies
6. Immune disorders
7. Hiatus hernia with gastro-oesophageal reflux

8. Cystic fibrosis – associated with failure to thrive ±
   malabsorption
9. Psychogenic cough – a well-recognized entity

Children with a persistent cough or a recurrent cough need
therefore a good assessment including a history, chest and ENT
examination and, as appropriate, CXR, RAST test, FBC and peak
flows. Asthma is very common and a trial of bronchodilator is
worthwhile, especially for those with recurrent coughs.

**THE WHEEZY CHILD**

1. Apart from asthma, the causes are viral or bacterial infection,
   anatomical anomalies (including laryngeal problems), inhaled
   foreign body and cystic fibrosis
2. In infants bronchiolitis, caused by respiratory syncytial virus
   (RSV), can cause wheeze
3. Various entities labelled, e.g. 'wheezy bronchitic', but they are
   largely academic as below the age of 2, where attacks of
   wheeze can be bought on by infection, bronchodilators are
   generally ineffective. A proportion of 'wheezy bronchitics' will
   develop asthma
4. Consider asthma in the child with recurrent cough,
   especially nocturnal cough, and in those with dyspnoea on
   exertion

**NOTES ON THE MANAGEMENT OF CHILDHOOD ASTHMA
(MAIN DISCUSSION OF ASTHMA IS IN THE MEDICAL CHAPTER)**

1. Take a full history
   (i) Atopy in the parents
   (ii) History of eczema, urticaria
   (iii) Nocturnal symptoms
   (iv) Relation of symptoms to exercise
   (v) Time off school
2. Examination – listen to the chest
3. Peak flow rate – parents can keep a record, especially for 'night
   coughers'
4. RAST test for allergies, e.g. house-dust mite. CXR if other
   suspected pathologies
5. Discussion with parents
   (i) Discussion generally about asthma – beware that 'asthma'
       is an emotive word to some
   (ii) Discussion on simple measures, especially against the
        house-dust mite
   (iii) Provision of a booklet explaining asthma and preventative
         measures
   (iv) Discussion of treatment

6. Treatment regimes
   These should follow the British Thoracic Society guidelines
   outlined on page 16
   For infrequent mild wheezy spells all that may be required is a
   β-adrenergic bronchodilator. For the child with frequent wheeze,
   time off school or recurrent attacks, Intal should be tried. Note that
   a trial of Intal requires regular use for at least 6–8 weeks. If Intal
   fails to control the asthma, inhaled steroids are the next step, e.g.
   beclomethasone (Becotide) or fluticasone (Flixotide). Fluticasone is
   licensed for children over 4 years of age.
7. Follow-up – ensure a follow-up system to monitor progress, i.e.
   frequency and severity of attacks, peak flows, time off school,
   treatment problems, etc.

## NOTES ON MANAGING THE CHILD WITH ABDOMINAL PAIN

1. Refresh yourself on traps for the unwary, i.e.
   intussusception, torsion of the testis, strangulated hernia and
   appendicitis
2. As a general rule regard acute abdominal pain as appendicitis
   until proved otherwise
3. Children may not have typical symptoms or signs – as always
   take a careful history, examine and test the urine
4. Remember to send off a urine culture if there is no obvious
   cause of the pain
5. Make arrangements to review the child unless obviously a
   benign gastroenteritis or mesenteric adenitis, and instruct the
   mother how and when to contact you
6. If you are unsure, ? appendicitis, ? mesenteric adenitis, it is best
   to refer. Mesenteric adenitis is favoured by a recent URTI and
   central rather than RIF tenderness
7. Recurrent abdominal pain affects 10% of schoolchildren
   but in less than 10% is a cause found. Look out for UTI and
   test and culture the urine in all. Rarer causes are peptic
   ulcers, Crohn's disease and food intolerance. More profitable
   is an exploration of the conflicts within the family and at
   school

## CHILD ABUSE

### History
1. Explanation inconsistent with the degree of injury
2. Discrepancies in the history
3. Delay in seeking medical help
4. Previous history of unexplained injury
5. Parental reaction one of over – or under-concern

6. Injury noted while examinining the child for another reason
7. Reluctance to allow examination of the child

## Examination
1. Torn frenulum of lip
2. Bites
3. Burns – especially cigarette burns
4. Bruising – especially circular bruises caused by fingertips, facial bruising (including black eyes), bruised ears, multiple bruising and bruises of different ages
5. Fractures
6. Signs of neglect – failure to thrive

## Management
1. Alert your health visitor and social worker
2. With anything other than trivial injury the best policy is to try and organize hospital admission (for documentation, clotting screen, skeletal survey, etc.)
3. Share responsibility with the social services. A case conference will be organized, which may return the child to the family with support and monitoring (the child having been placed on the At-Risk Register) or, in more severe cases, an application may be made to the Juvenile Court for a care order

## DEVELOPMENTAL SURVEILLANCE

As part of the 1990 Contract, suitably trained GPs will receive a capitation fee supplement for every child under 5 years of age registered with them for the surveillance service. Health Authorities will maintain a list of GPs eligible to provide the service in their area – the Child Health Surveillance List.

Practices will therefore be looking to set up a system of child health clinics to provide this service. This will entail:
1. Discussion between the partners and the health visitors over the time and place of the paediatric surveillance and the role of each team member
2. Adoption of a recall and record storage system (based inevitably on a computerized system)
3. Familiarization with the local health authority programme (and liaison with local community paediatricians)
4. Further training to achieve the required eligibility for the Child Health Surveillance List
5. Purchase of the following equipment and books (reproduced with permission, form Mead  1989 *How to set up a Child Health Clinic*, Update 39: 400):

- Percentile charts
- Child health record cards
- Measuring instruments
  - scales for infants
  - scales for older children
  - wall measuring chart
  - tape measures
- High frequency rattle
- Cup and spoon
- MEG warbler (device that emits specific sounds)
- Balls, Smarties and 'hundreds and thousands'
- Bag full of at least twelve 1-inch brick cubes in various colours
- Series of picture cards
- Box full of toys for distraction testing
- Full set of Stycar charts and test cards

1. GMSC/Royal College of General Practitioners. *Handbook of preventative care for pre-school children.* London: Royal College of General Practitioners, 1988
2. Hall D (ed). *Health for all children. A programme for child surveillance.* Oxford: Oxford University Press, 1989
3. Lingam S, Harvey D. *Manual of child development.* Edinburgh: Churchill Livingstone, 1988

Note that:
1. Child health clinics are a good opportunity not only for developmental assessments but also for discussion of mother's worries on a wide range of problems (feeding, crying, rashes etc.) and for the promotion of immunization
2. Percentile charts are an essential part of paediatric care and all GPs should have the full range
3. It is important to have a knowledge of the major milestone e.g. sits with no support between 6 and 8 months, pulls to stand at 10 months, etc. Infants should double their birth weight by 5 months and treble it in a year. As a general rule children are half their adult height by 2 years, dry by day at 2 years and dry by night at 3 years
4. There are lots of different tests and procedures but the crucial and well-validated areas that must not be missed are congenital dislocation of the hip, undescended testes, squint and vision defects, hearing defects and scoliosis. The health visitor should also check that the neonatal screen for phenylketonuria and hypothyroidism has been carried out
5. The stages for screening will be
   - at birth
   - 6 weeks
   - 8 months (range 7–9 months)
   - 21 months (range 18–24 months)
   - 39 months (range 36–42 months)
   Some of these checks will be chiefly the responsibility of the GP (e.g. the 6-week check) and some more the responsibility of

the health visitor (e.g. the 8-month check). As an example of a check, consider the 6-week check

## The 6-week check
1. Record weight, height and head circumference and plot on a centile chart
2. General examination as at birth but especially eyes (? red reflex, ? following), heart (congenital heart disease in 6/1000 births), femoral pulses, hernial orifices, testes to see if descended, hips to exclude dislocation (but easier to detect in the newborn), lower limbs (? talipes) and spine
3. Check developmental milestones at 6 weeks
   (i) Motor
      a. Test head lag – should be still marked but not complete
      b. Prone – may just transiently lift head off the couch
      c. Ventral suspension – head can be held level with trunk
      d. Moro reflex – should be symmetrical
   (ii) Hearing – does baby respond to sound ?
   (iii) Vision – eyes can fixate and follow moving persons
   (iv) Social – is baby smiling ?
4. Discuss and promote immunization
5. Discuss feeding and any other problems with the mother

## Other checks
For details of the other checks see the references listed above

# Immunization

Table 9 The current standard immunization schedule for children

| Age | Immunization |
|---|---|
| 2 months | 1st triple* + polio. Hib vaccine |
| 3 months | 2nd triple + polio. Hib vaccine |
| 4 months | 3rd triple + polio. Hib vaccine |
| 12–18 months | Measles/Mumps/Rubella (MMR vaccine) |
| 4½–5 years (pre-school booster) | Dip/Tet + polio |
| 10–14 years | Rubella (for girls only who haven't received MMR vaccine) |
| 10–14 years | BCG (to tuberculin-negative children) |
| 15–18 years (school leavers) | Tetanus + polio |

*The triple refers, of course, to the Dlp/Tet/Pertussis vaccine.
Hib = Haemophilus influenzae type B

## CONTRAINDICATIONS TO THE VACCINES

### General contraindications to live vaccines (MMR, polio, BCG)
1. Pregnancy
2. Any acute febrile illness – not just a snuffly cold
3. Patients who are immunosuppressed or receiving radiotherapy
4. Patients with malignant conditions (including leukaemia and lymphomas)
5. Patients on steroids
6. Within 3 weeks of receiving another live vaccine

## Diphtheria

Not to be given over the age of 10 years without a Schick test, to those with a previous serious reaction to the vaccine or those with an acute infection

## Tetanus

*Contraindications*

A booster should not be given routinely if the patient has had a tetanus vaccination within the previous year. Also, not to those with a previous serious reaction to the vaccine or those with an acute infection

*Practical notes*
1. The dose of dip/tet or tetanus vaccine is 0.5 ml either by s.c. or i.m. injection
2. The main side-effect of both is local swelling and redness at the site of the injection

## Polio

*Contraindications*
1. General contraindications to live vaccines as above
2. Not to be given if diarrhoea and vomiting
3. Not to be given if severe hypersensitivity to penicillin, neomycin, polymyxin or streptomycin – but manufacturers stress that the minute traces of penicillin should not normally contraindicate unless the hypersensitivity is extreme

*Practical notes*
1. Give orally – drops to babies, on a sugar lump in older children
2. Breastfeeding not a contraindication
3. Extremely remote risk of vaccine-related paralysis in unvaccinated contacts (about 1 in 2.5 million risk) and thus polio vaccine should also be offered to unvaccinated parents and siblings at the same time

## Pertussis (whooping cough)

*Contraindications*
1. Children with a history of severe local or general reaction to a preceding dose (not just local erythema and swelling) is the only true contraindication. If the child has an acute febrile illness, immunization should be postponed
   Rather than refuse pertussis vaccination, certain children need a more detailed consideration before the vaccine is given. Discussion with a paediatrician would be appropriate in the following cases:

(i)  where the child has previously had a convulsion or an apnoeic attack
(ii)  where there is a first-degree relative (parents or siblings) with epilepsy. Current DHSS advice is to confine the consideration of epilepsy to the parents and siblings of the child. Even then the risk is very small
(iii)  children who have had brain damage in the neonatal period

*Practical notes*
1. The risk of pertussis vaccine causing persisting neurological damage was estimated to be 1 in 300 000 injections by the National  Childhood Encephalopathy Study (1981)
2. A history of allergy, asthma or eczema is *not* a contraindication
3. Warn patients of possible irritability and mild temperature that evening and to give a dose of Calpol in his instance
4. Usually given as part of the triple (dip/tet/pertussis) but can be given separately

**Measles/Mumps/Rubella (MMR) vaccine**

*Contraindications*
1. General contraindications to live vaccines, as above
2. Active tuberculosis
3. Hypersensitivity to neomycin or kanamycin
4. Blood dyscrasias such as thrombocytopenia
5. Within 3 months of an injection of immunoglobulin
6. Anaphylactoid reaction to eggs (i.e. urticaria, mouth swelling, etc. – not just a dislike of eggs!)
7. Children under 1 year of age – ineffective due to the presence of passive antibodies from the mother

*Practical notes*
1. Every year children die of measles, a few children develop a subacute sclerosing panencephalitis as a complication and 1 in 1000 cases of measles develops an encephalitis – it is not a benign disease
2. Chance of permanent damage due to the vaccine, estimated at about 1 in a million vaccinations
3. Dose is 0.5 ml i.m. or s.c.
4. A mild measles-like illness may occur about the eighth day after vaccination and rarely a parotid swelling appears about the third week
5. Children with fits or a family history of fits *should be* vaccinated – with advice re temperature reduction and management of a fit

6. History of measles, mumps or rubella is no contraindication
7. Children are not infectious post vaccination
8. If no record of MMR, vaccination should also be given to children aged 4–5 years before starting school
9. Can be given together with other vaccines (in the opposite arm)

## Rubella (German measles)

*Contraindications*
1. General contraindications to live vaccines as above
2. Pregnancy the obvious one – but hardly likely in the children being considered. Remember if vaccinating others or postpartum, that pregnancy must be avoided for at least 3 months
3. Hypersensitivity to neomycin
4. Children with thrombocytopenia
5. Within 3 months of a blood transfusion (interference from passive antibodies) or human immune serum globulin

*Practical notes*
1. The dose is 0.5 ml s.c.
2. Ignore any history of possible rubella in the past – unreliable
3. Side-effects uncommon but include transient rash, lymphadenopathy, arthralgia and very, very rarely, thrombocytopenia

## BCG

*Contraindications*
1. General contraindications to live vaccines as above
2. Generalized infective dermatoses. Eczema itself not a contraindication, providing vaccination given in lesion-free skin
3. Local sepsis
4. HIV infection

*Practical notes*
1. Given to tuberculin-negative children
2. No live vaccine to be given for at least 3 weeks after BCG vaccination and none in the same arm for 3 months (risk of regional lymphadenopathy)
3. Can be given to neonates (providing mothers have not received antenatal steroid therapy)
4. Important to give BCG vaccination at birth to babies of immigrants from countries where tuberculosis common
5. Use the intradermal preparation for babies making sure it is given intradermally, NOT subcutaneously

### Hib (Haemophilus influenzae b)

*Contraindications*
1. Acute illness (not a snuffly cold) — in which case postpone
2. Previous severe reaction to Hib. Hib is given with the triple and any adverse reaction will probably be from the triple rather than Hib

*Practical notes*
1. Not a live vaccine
2. Hib itself can cause meningitis, epiglottitis and septicaemia. Worth protecting against
3. Children under 13 months should receive 3 doses, those between 13 and 48 months a single dose
4. Vaccine can be used to immunize contacts of Hib disease under 4 years of age (infection uncommon after 4)

## PROCEDURE AT THE IMMUNIZATION CLINIC

1. Often conducted with the health visitors
2. Check availability of up-to-date ampoules of 1 in 1000 adrenaline in case of a severe anaphylactic reaction
3. Explain the procedure to the mother and make sure consent has been obtained
4. Check with the mother on the contraindications to the proposed immunization
5. Check on current health of the child – note that a simple snuffly cold would not be a contraindication
6. Carry out the immunization procedure
7. Warn of the possible side-effects (Calpol for temperature, mild measles – like illness in 8 days, etc.)
8. Ensure you have entered the immunization on the child's record

## TARGET PAYMENT SYSTEM FOR CHILDHOOD IMMUNIZATION

### A. Children aged 2 and under

1. There are four groups of immunizations for children aged 2 and under

Group 1: Diphtheria/Tetanus and Polio. 3 doses complete the course

Group 2: Pertussis. 3 doses complete the course

Group 3: Measles/Mumps/Rubella (MMR) or measles vaccine alone. One dose

Group 4: Hib vaccine. 3 doses complete the course or the over 13 months single dose

Only complete courses will count towards your target, i.e. all

3 doses must have been given if 3 doses complete the course.

2. There are two target levels – 90% and 70%. On the first day of each quarter you will be eligible for payment if you have achieved an average of 70% coverage level of the number of complete courses required to fully immunize all the children aged 2 on your list on that particular day. By taking average coverage levels you can compensate for a lower than 70% coverage in one group (e.g. Pertussis) by a higher than 70% coverage in another group (e.g. MMR vaccine). For example:

   Suppose a GP has a target population of 20 children aged 2 on his list.

   Suppose 16 have received complete course of Dip/Tet and Polio
   　　　　12 have received complete courses of Pertussis
   　　　　14 have received the MMR vaccine
   　　　　14 received complete courses of Hib vaccination

   For 20 children the number of complete courses to fully immunize = 80 (each child requiring 4 complete courses)
   Number actually given = $16 + 12 + 14 + 14 = 56 = 56/80 = 70\%$.
   The 70% target payment has been achieved, even though the pertussis level achieved was lower than this

3. Calculation of the exact payment. This will depend on three factors:
   (i) The target level achieved – the ratio of payment is to be 3:1 in favour of the higher 90% target
   (ii) The number of children on the list i.e. the more children on the list the higher the payment
   (iii) The percentage of immunizations actually given by the GP. If a DHA clinic does some of the immunizations, for example, the GP's payment is correspondingly reduced. Note that it is the GP giving the third and final immunization in a group who will be credited with the course

## B. Pre-school boosters for children aged 5 and under
An identical system will operate for the Dip/Tet and Polio vaccination given pre-school

## INFLUENZA VACCINATION

1. Recommended for those patients
   (i) With chronic pulmonary disease, e.g. chronic bronchitis, asthma
   (ii) With chronic heart disease
   (iii) With chronic renal disease
   (iv) With diabetes mellitus

(v) Who are elderly and living in situations where the risk of spread is high (residential homes, nursing homes, etc.)
2. Contraindicated in those hypersensitive to egg and chicken protein

## HEPATITIS B VACCINATION (ENGERIX B)

1. In three doses provides over 90% protection against hepatitis B infection
2. Can be prescribed on an FP10 as Engerix B
3. Recommended for various high-risk groups, i.e.
    (i) Dentists and dental technicians and assistants
    (ii) Doctors, nurses and any health care personnel at risk of exposure (e.g. handling blood products)
    (iii) Those treated by haemodialysis or requiring frequent blood transfusions
    (iv) Residents and staff of mental institutions
    (v) Homosexuals
    (vi) Prostitutes
    (vii) Those who abuse drugs
    (viii) Partners of patients with active hepatitis B or carriers
    (ix) Some would extend the list to include police, prison and ambulance personnel
4. Regimen is three doses by intramuscular injection, second dose 1 month after the first and third dose 5 months after the second
5. Screening can be carried out 4 months after the course to see if there has been an appropriate antibody response. If not consider a booster. The duration of protection is believed to be at least 5 years

## HEPATITIS A VACCINATION (HAVRIX)

1. Inactivated vaccine. Two doses intramuscularly in the deltoid spaced 2 weeks – 1 month apart gives antibodies for a year. A third dose 6–12 months after the initial dose provides immunity for up to 10 years. A Havrix Monodose is now available
2. Can be given simultaneously with human normal immunoglobulin (at a different site)
3. There is a junior vaccine for those aged 1–15 years
4. Particularly recommended for frequent travellers and those spending more than 3 months abroad

## VACCINATIONS FOR TRAVELLING

1. Encourage patients to plan ahead as early as possible

2. Consult the schedules in *Pulse or Doctor* for the latest recommendations
3. Prior to vaccination check patient is well and there are no contraindications (on steroids, immunosuppressed, pregnant, etc.)

**Standard course for travel**
Assuming not previously immunized, the course would be:
Typhoid (inactivated), cholera + tetanus + polio
then 6 weeks later:
2nd typhoid (inactivated) 2nd cholera, 2nd tetanus + 2nd dose polio
On return, 6 months after the 2nd dose, the polio and tetanus courses can be completed. If already immunized against polio and tetanus may need just a booster dose, but will not even need a booster if had a 3rd dose or booster within last 5 years
*Note*: Typhim Vi is a single dose inactivated typhoid vaccine.

**Rabies**
A human diploid cell vaccine is available for those at great risk, e.g. vets

**γ-Globulin for hepatitis A prevention (if given instead of HAVRIX)**
Do not give before a polio vaccination or less than 3 weeks after, as it may interfere with the immune response. Doubtful whether γ-globulin interferes with yellow fever vaccination significantly but the same advice often given for yellow fever, i.e. do not give γ-globulin before or less than 3 weeks after

**Yellow fever**
1. Can be given simultaneously with polio but if this has already been given, you need to wait 3 weeks before giving the polio
2. Hence given first in the series. Does not interfere with any killed vaccine

**Malaria**
1. Consult *Pulse's 'Foreign Travel Guide'* which is updated monthly
2. Remember
   (i) Malaria can be contacted on stopovers – even while the plane is on the tarmac at a foreign airport
   (ii) To start prophylaxis 1 week before and to continue for 4 weeks after returning
   (iii) To give children as well as adults prophylaxis

**Vaccination in a hurry**
1. Cholera and typhoid (inactivated) can be given with a 4-week interval between. If less time, the two doses of cholera can be

**Table 10**

| Vaccination | Lasts | Dose for course | Interval between 1st & 2nd dose | Notes |
|---|---|---|---|---|
| Typhoid (inactivated vaccine) | 3 years | 1st: >10 years, 0.5 ml s.c./i.m. 1–10 years, 0.25 ml s.c./i.m. <1 year, not recommended | 4–6 weeks Booster every 3 years | Gives 70–80% protection Also a single dose vaccine available (Typhim Vi). |
| Typhoid (live vaccine = Vivotif) | 3 years | 2nd: 0.1 ml by intradermal injection Oral: 3 capsules on alternate days (days 1, 3 and 5) | | Rules for live vaccines apply. Interacts with antibiotics and mefloquine (see literalure) |
| Cholera | 6 months | 1st: 1–5 years, 0.1 ml s.c/i.m. 5–10 years, 0.3 ml s.c./i.m. >10 years, 0.5 ml s.c./i.m. <1 year, not recommended  2nd: 1–10 years 0.1 ml intradermal >10 years 0.2 ml intradermal | 4–6 weeks Booster every 6 months or longer | Protection probably only 50%. Only one injection required for the International Certificate, which becomes valid 6 days after first dose of vaccine |
| Yellow fever | 10 years | One injection of live attenuated vaccine arranged at a special centre | | Very effective. International Certificate valid for 10 years from the 10th day after vaccination (hence must go at least 10 days before travelling) |

given with 7 days between and one typhoid (inactivated) vaccination will protect for 6 months (no need for an International Certificate with typhoid)
2. A booster tetanus and polio can be given at the same time as typhoid and cholera
3. Remember malaria prophylaxis!

**Payment**
1. Health authorities will pay for some recommended vaccinations, including the booster polio and tetanus
2. Can charge a fee for the International Cholera Certificate

# Infectious diseases

**MEASLES**

Incubation period 10–15 days

**Period for which patient infectious**
From prodromal symptoms 4–5 days before rash until 5 days after onset of the rash

**Clinical features aiding diagnosis**
Starts as a coryzal illness with harsh cough, running eyes and fever. Kopliks spots (like grains of salt on the buccal mucosa) appear about 2 days later and on about fourth day a red maculopapular rash appears behind the ears spreading to face and trunk, coalescing to form blotchy patches

*Notes:*
1. Cough is a characteristic feature and often associated with signs in chest
2. If temperature not settling within a few days of the rash appearing suspect secondary infection

**Complications**
1. Otitis media (commonest)
2. Chest infection (but cough part of illness)
3. Conjunctivitis
4. Febrile convulsions with fever
5. Gastroenteritis
6. Laryngeal stridor
7. Encephalitis in 1:1000. Many years after an attack a risk of subacute sclerosing panencephalitis

**Management**
Antibiotics useful for otitis media and chest infection but not for routine prophylaxis. Chloramphenicol eye drops for conjunctivitis

## RUBELLA (GERMAN MEASLES)

Incubation period 14–21 days

**Period for which patient infectious**
From 7 days prior to rash until 5 days after

**Clinical features aiding diagnosis**
May be a mild viral illness, perhaps with a pharyngitis and lymphadenopathy – especially the suboccipital nodes. A pink macular rash appears on face first, spreading rapidly over trunk and lasting 2–3 days at the most. However, patient may be well and afebrile. Rash may be fleeting or absent. It is rarely possible to make a definite diagnosis on clinical grounds – many cases are totally asymptomatic

**Complications**
Arthralgia may occur in adolescents and adults. Other complications (thrombocytopenia and encephalitis) extremely rare

**Management**
No treatment. If patient is pregnant and there is suggestion of a contact with rubella, do serial blood tests to detect a recent infection

## CHICKENPOX

Incubation period 11–21 days

**Period for which patient infectious**
From 2 days before rash develops until 7 days after the last crop

**Clinical features aiding diagnosis**
Rash appears as first sign of illness, appearing in crops mainly on the trunk. Lesions go through macular, papular, vesicular and pustular stages before drying to form scabs. Often lesions in the mouth

**Complications and management**
Encephalitis with cerebellar involvement a rare complication, as is pneumonia. Lesions may become secondarily infected in which case prescribe flucloxacillin. Otherwise use calamine lotion for the

spots. Acyclovir (Zovirax) is now licensed for the treatment of chickenpox and may be considered for severer cases

## MUMPS
Incubation period 12–28 days

### Period for which patient infectious
From 3 days prior to the swelling until 7 days after it resolves

### Clinical features aiding diagnosis
May be mild prodromal symptoms prior to swelling of salivary glands. Parotid glands nearly always affected, sometimes unilaterally and may also affect submandibular glands

### Complications and management
Aseptic meningitis common but usually mild and manageable at home. Orchitis, rare before puberty, usually unilateral and rarely, if ever, causes infertility. Oophoritis, pancreatitis and encephalitis all very rare complications

## PERTUSSIS (WHOOPING COUGH)
Incubation period 7–10 days

### Period for which patient infectious
From 2 days prior to start of symptoms, until up to 5 weeks after the onset of the cough

### Clinical features aiding diagnosis
A catarrhal stage precedes the paroxysmal stage. Cough is
1. Paroxysmal – spasms with possible cyanosis ending in a whoop
2. Often associated with vomiting
3. Persistent for weeks or months (the '100-day' cough). Infants may have no whoop but present as apnoeic/cyanotic spells. Pernasal swab not a practical method of diagnosis

### Complications
1. Cerebral – fits, hemiplegia encephalopathy. A few (mainly < 6 months old) die
2. Respiratory – bronchopneumonia, lobar collapse

### Management
1. Symptomatic – tube feeding, oxygen, etc., in severe cases

2. Erythromycin for 14 days to patient and non-immune infant contacts said by some to reduce infectivity of pertussis

## SHINGLES

1. Caused by reactivation of varicella zoster (chickenpox) virus
2. Characteristically pain precedes the vesicular eruption in the dermatome
3. Post-herpetic neuralgia can be severe – try co-proxamol plus a low dose of amitriptyline at night
4. A child can catch chickenpox from visiting her grandmother with shingles but the reverse is said not to occur
5. In the acute stage use either acyclovir (Zovirax) 800 mg five times a day for 7 days or famciclovir (Famvir) three times daily for 7 days. Must start treatment within 72 hrs of rash.

## COLD SORES (HERPES SIMPLEX)

If started at first sign of developing a cold sore, acyclovir (Zovirax) cream five times a day for 5 days is effective

## NOTIFIABLE DISEASES

Common diseases notifiable to district community physician (a fee is payed for each notification) are:
Acute encephalitis
Dysentery – amoebic/bacillary
Food poisoning
Leptospirosis
Malaria
Measles
Meningitis (also meningococcal septicaemia without meningitis)
Mumps
Rubella
Scarlet fever
Tuberculosis
Viral hepatitis
Whooping cough
Plus a few of the rarer infections you will never see – should you do so, check the book! Note that AIDS is not yet a statutory notifiable disease

## DIARRHOEA

For childhood diarrhoea *see* Paediatric chapter. For adult diarrhoea, the plan is shown in Table 11

**Table 11**

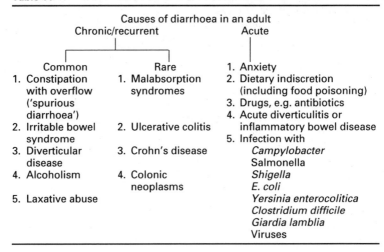

Causes of diarrhoea in an adult

| Chronic/recurrent | | Acute |
|---|---|---|
| Common | Rare | 1. Anxiety |
| 1. Constipation with overflow ('spurious diarrhoea') | 1. Malabsorption syndromes | 2. Dietary indiscretion (including food poisoning) |
| | | 3. Drugs, e.g. antibiotics |
| | | 4. Acute diverticulitis or inflammatory bowel disease |
| 2. Irritable bowel syndrome | 2. Ulcerative colitis | 5. Infection with |
| 3. Diverticular disease | 3. Crohn's disease | *Campylobacter* |
| | | *Salmonella* |
| 4. Alcoholism | 4. Colonic neoplasms | *Shigella* |
| | | *E. coli* |
| 5. Laxative abuse | | *Yersinia enterocolitica* |
| | | *Clostridium difficile* |
| | | *Giardia lamblia* |
| | | Viruses |

## Assessment
1. Length of history
2. Recent dietary indiscretion?
3. Contacts with symptoms?
4. Recent foreign travel?
5. Frequency and consistency of stools – any blood?
6. Work – ? food-handler
7. Any vomiting?

## Examination
1. Is patient dehydrated?
2. Is abdomen soft?

## Stool culture
Only worth it if
1. Patient handles food as part of work
2. Persistent, severe or bloody diarrhoea
3. Diarrhoea in an institution
4. Suspected food poisoning
5. Patient has recently travelled abroad
6. A treatable cause is expected, i.e.
   (i) Diarrhoea after antibiotics (? pseudomembranous colitis caused by *Clostridium difficile* and treated by metronidazole)
   (ii) *Campylobacter*, which presents as cramps and profuse,

often bloody diarrhoea and is treated by erythromycin
500 mg qds for 7 days
(iii)  Giardiasis, where the diarrhoea resembles a steatorrhoea
and the treatment is metronidazole

**Treatment**
1. Treat dehydration, e.g. using Dioralyte sachets
2. Antidiarrhoeals, e.g. loperamide (Imodium) 4 mg stat, then a
   2-mg capsule after each loose stool, up to eight capsules a day
3. Treatable causes as above. In acute travellers' diarrhoea,
   ciprofloxacin (ciproxin) is worth a try. *Salmonella* and *Shigella*
   not treated unless the severe bacteraemic form is encountered
4. Advice – general advice about avoiding food, etc.

# Gynaecology

## VAGINAL DISCHARGE

*Causes*
1. Physiological – premenstrual, at ovulation, pregnancy
2. Infections
    (i) Secondary to a cervicitis caused by *Neisseria gonorrhoeae*, herpes simplex or *Chlamydia trachomatis*
    (ii) True vaginal infections – *Candida albicans, Trichomonas vaginalis* and *Gardnerella vaginalis*
3. Foreign body/retained tampon
4. Cervical polyps
5. Neoplasms of the cervix or uterine body
6. Sensitivity to chemicals (disinfectants, antiseptics, etc.)

**Management**
1. Unrealistic to investigate all fully
2. At least one-third will have classical *Candida* infection with pruritus and/or a creamy discharge
    Suggested scheme of management is shown in Table 12

**Practical notes**
1. Review cervical cytology status – if no recent smear, take one
2. If male partner has urethritis, suspect *Chlamydia* or *Neisseria*
3. *Chlamydia* is an important cause of infection and infertility – difficult to diagnose in general practice, so refer if cervicitis or urethritis in the partner
4. With a microscope it is possible to identify *Trichomonas* directly by examining the discharge in a drop of saline
5. Key difficulty is the possibility of sexually transmitted disease (STD). Keep this possibility in the back of your mind
6. If no suspected STD, no cervicitis, no symptoms in the partner, no local lesion or abdominal pain, then effectively the treatment is either antifungal or metronidazole 400 mg bd for 5 days

**Table 12**

Patient presents with a vaginal discharge

Ask about colour, consistency, odour, blood-staining, symptoms in the partner, associated pain. Is the discharge recurrent?

| White creamy discharge + pruritus | Inoffensive, non-itchy, clear discharge | Offensive smell, greenish/yellow, blood-stained, associated abdominal pain, symptoms in partner, recurrent |
|---|---|---|
| Treat as probable *Candida*, investigating if not resolving on treatment | Probably physiological | If any of the above symptoms or signs |
| | Assess menstrual symptoms, LMP, use of the pill | |
| | Examine to reassure the patient | |
| | | Speculum examination |

| Foreign body or tampon | Cervical polyp | No polyp or foreign body |
|---|---|---|
| Remove | Refer | |

| Associated abdominal pain | Suspected cervical infection or sexually transmitted disease | Discharge in the vagina |
|---|---|---|
| Vaginal examination and swabs for *Neisseria* and *Chlamydia*. Difficulty in taking these in general practice may necessitate referral. If neither swabs nor immediate referral possible, treat with erythromycin 250 mgs and metronidazole 400 mg bd for 2 weeks. With abdominal pain as a symptom, make absolutely sure patient is not pregnant | Refer to genito-urinary clinic for swabs and contact tracing | Take an HVS and charcoal swab, if appropriate |
| | | While waiting swabs, treat for *Trichomonas* and *Gardnerella*, assuming no *Candida* found – both respond to metronidazole 400 mg bd for 5 days (also treat partner) |
| If not referred, review | | Review with results NB gonorrhoea can coexist with *Trichomonas* |

**Treatment of candidiasis**
1. First attack or infrequent attacks – use pessaries and cream (e.g. Canesten) or tampons (Gyno-Daktarin). Treat partner with cream
2. Recurrent
   (i) Exclude diabetes mellitus and iron deficiency
   (ii) Advice – avoid tights, wear cotton pants, wash with plain soap and water daily, avoid vaginal deodorants
   (iii) Make sure partner has been treated
   (iv) Intermittent use of tampons or pessaries or longer courses, remembering not to stop around the time of the period, e.g. use of Canesten 1 (single clotrimazole pessary with applicator) once a week for 4–5 weeks or monthly just after a period for a few months
   (v) Oral therapy with nystatin to eradicate the bowel reservoir
   (vi) Use of natural yoghurt (or lactic acid pessaries) put into the vagina at the first indication of an attack or prior to menstruation may be useful in aborting some episodes
   (vii) Use of single capsule therapy with fluconazole (Diflucan). Expensive, but very useful for the treatment of recurrent candidiasis. Beware drug interactions

## THE MENOPAUSE
1. Average age in the UK is 51 years. There is a 2–3-year period (the climacteric) during which reproductive function ceases and ovarian hormones decline
2. Symptoms of climacteric and menopause include vasomotor symptoms (flushes and sweats), urinary symptoms (due to atrophic changes – may cause frequency and dysuria), atrophic vaginitis and psychological symptoms (some due to the vasomotor symptoms and insomnia). Osteoporosis is a long-term result of oestrogen deficiency
3. Contraception is needed for 2 years after the last menstrual period
4. Postmenopausal bleeding (bleeding 6 months after the LMP) needs referral for a D & C/hysteroscopy

## HORMONE REPLACEMENT THERAPY (HRT)

**Indications**
1. Vasomotor symptoms, atrophic vaginitis and atrophic urethritis
2. Debateable use for psychological symptoms – some would try but many say main effect on psychological symptoms is a placebo one

3. There is a case for long-term (> 5 years) HRT to prevent fractures due to osteoporosis
4. Local dienoestrol cream and lubricant jelly may be the sole therapy for senile vaginitis – contraindications for dienoestrol cream same as for HRT
5. Those with a premature menopause (natural or surgically induced) should be offered HRT

*Note*: HRT also reduces the risk of coronary heart disease

## Contraindications

*Absolute*
1. Endometrial carcinoma
2. Carcinoma of breast
3. Abnormal vaginal bleeding needs investigation prior to HRT
4. Pregnancy
5. Severe liver disease
6. Otosclerosis

*Notes:*
1. Since HRT will reduce cardiovascular disease risk it can be prescribed to those with hypertension (but monitor) or ischaemic heart disease. Similarly it can be given to smokers or diabetics
2. Relative contraindications include fibroids and gall bladder disease
3. The increased risk of breast cancer with HRT is related to duration of use – negligible risk if used for 5 years or less

## Treatment regimen
1. Choice of treatment. If patient has had a hysterectomy, continuous oestrogen, starting with the lowest dose, with tablets (e.g. Premarin, Progynova) an implant, or transdermal oestrogen patches. If uterus present there is a danger of endometrial hyperplasia and carcinoma, hence use cyclical oestrogen – progestogen preparations (e.g. CycloProgynova)
2. Initial assessment
   (i) Check contraindications
   (ii) Check weight, BP and breasts
   (iii) Ask about any abnormal vaginal bleeding. Check date of last smear and perform a pelvic examination (? fibroids, ? ovarian cyst, etc.)
3. Follow-up
   (i) 6-monthly BP check
   (ii) Annual breast and pelvic examination
   (iii) Encourage breast self-examination and ensure smears are up to date
   (iv) Refer any unexpected or irregular vaginal bleeding

4. Duration of treatment. Try weaning off after 2 years, reducing the dose slowly over 3 months. Some need longer. For prevention of osteoporosis, see literature

## THE INFERTILE COUPLE

### Definition
Failure to conceive within a year of unprotected intercourse (at least twice a week)

### Male
1. Take a history of previous testicular problems, smoking and alcohol
2. Exclude a varicocele
3. Arrange a sperm count – a specimen after 3 days abstinence from intercourse
   Normal sperm count: Volume > 2 ml
   Sperm count > 20 million/ml
   Motility > 60% of sperms
   Abnormal forms < 40%

### Female
1. Take a full history (previous obstetric, gynaecological and menstrual history)
2. Examination, including pelvic examination
3. Instruct patient in the filling-in of a temperature chart

### Couple
Enquire about frequency of intercourse, specific sexual problems (e.g. premature ejaculation) and general fears and worries
After the above assessment the GP should be in a good position to offer advice and refer to the appropriate specialist for help

## PREMENSTRUAL TENSION

Variety of symptoms including depression (suicide commoner premenstrually), irritability, headache, feelings of bloatedness, mastalgia, etc.

### Management
1. Sympathy, reassurance and support
2. Progestogen therapy either orally (dydrogesterone 10 mg bd from days 12 to 26) or by pessaries/suppositories (Cyclogest 200 mg or 400 mg from the 12th or 14th day until menstruation)
3. Pyridoxine 50 mg bd from 14th day of the cycle
4. Diuretics for the premenstrual week – often unhelpful

5. For younger patients, consider the oral contraceptive pill
6. If all else fails, consider trying danazol (Danol)

**Notes**
1. Exclude a true depression (better treated by antidepressants, etc.)
2. Keeping of a menstrual calendar useful in diagnosing truly premenstrual symptoms and in monitoring progress

## DYSMENORRHOEA

For primary dysmenorrhoea the choices are mefenamic acid (Ponstan) 500 mg tds from the onset of menstrual pain, dydrogesterone (Duphaston) 10 mg bd from days 5 to 25 or the oral contraceptive pill

## HEAVY OR IRREGULAR MENSTRUAL LOSS

**Causes**
Pregnancy, miscarriage, retained products of conception
The IUCD
Polyps
Fibroids
Pelvic inflammatory disease
Carcinoma of the cervix or endometrium
Endometriosis
Blood dyscrasias
Hypothyroidism
'Dysfunctional uterine bleeding' – including anovulatory bleeding (at menarche or menopause) and ovulatory bleeding
Psychological causes

**Management**
1. History, including contraception and LMP
2. Examination (VE and speculum) plus cervical smear
3. If menorrhagia, an FBC
    < 35 years old – if no obvious cause and the bleeding persists longer than 3 months consider:
    (i) The oral contraceptive pill
    (ii) Mefenamic acid (Ponstan) 500 mg tds for 5 days starting at menstruation (useful for IUCD bleeding)
    (iii) Anovulatory cycles may respond to norethisterone (Primolut N)
    (iv) If all else fails danazol 100–400 mg daily, but ensure contraception is used
    > 35 years old and no obvious cause:
    (i) A diagnostic curettage/hysteroscopy should be considered

to exclude a carcinoma of the endometrium, especially
with heavy or irregular bleeding around the menopause
(ii) Try norethisterone (Primolut N) – see literature
(iii) A short course of danazol can be tried but side-effects
(weight gain, etc.) may be a problem
(iv) If a D & C is negative, norethisterone fails and the
menopause is not imminent, consider hysterectomy

**Notes**
1. Remember oral iron if anaemic
2. For irregular bleeding, especially in a patient > 35 years, refer
for assessment. For patients < 35 years with heavy, regular
bleeding a D & C is rarely helpful, either therapeutically or
diagnostically

# Cervical cytology

## INTRODUCTION

There is thought to be a gradation thus:

Mild dysplasia → Moderate → Severe dysplasia/ → Invasive
                 dysplasia    carcinoma in situ    carcinoma
(CIN 1)          (CIN 2)      (CIN 3)

*Notes:*
1. Some cases of dysplasia can revert to normal
2. There appears to be a more aggressive form, especially in younger women, with rapid change from normal cervix to carcinoma

## STATISTICS

1. Each year over 2000 women die in the UK from carcinoma of the cervix
2. Incidence of carcinoma of the cervix is increasing in young women, although still only about 5% of deaths occur under 35 years

## HIGH-RISK GROUPS

1. Those with factors related to sexual activity viz:
   (i) Early first coitus
   (ii) Sexually transmitted disease
   (iii) Many sexual partners
2. Those with a history of genital warts or whose partner has penile warts (since a human papilloma virus may play an important role in the pathogenesis)
3. Those in lower socio-economic groups – many factors may be operating here
4. Smokers – cervical carcinoma has a higher incidence in smokers

*Note:* Cervical carcinoma is increasingly regarded as a sexually transmitted disease and, just as with AIDS, barrier methods of contraception are protective

## THE CERVICAL CYTOLOGY SCREENING PROGRAMME

1. Over the last few years Health Authorities have introduced computerized recall systems for all patients due a smear. The routine screening programme in most areas of the country will run as follows:
   - GPs are sent a list of those due a smear to check before the patient is called
   - the GP returns the checked list: patients who have had a hysterectomy including removal of the cervix should be notified so that they can be excluded from the programme
   - the Health Authority calls the patients using the corrected list. If there is still no record of a smear after 6 months from the initial invitation, the patient is sent a reminder letter. If still no response the GP is sent a 'non-responder' card to put in the medical records
2. The current guidelines are to take smears of women aged 20–64. Screening is also advised at the onset of sexual activity and during early pregnancy. The precise recall system in operation will vary slightly from area to area – in Leicestershire the Health Authority recalls women aged 18–44 every 3 years and women aged 45–65 every 5 years
3. Those with abnormal smears will need more frequent follow-up. It is also advisable to screen yearly women with genital warts (or whose partners have anal or genital warts)
4. Opportunistic screening of 'non-responders' and women in high-risk groups who are overdue or have never had a smear is vital to the success of the fight against cervical cancer
5. It is essential to have an efficient system for referring/following up those patients with abnormal smears, rather than totally relying on the computerized system

## TAKING THE SMEAR

1. A technique to be learnt
2. Make sure you scrape the cervix through a complete 360° and that the smear is immediately covered with fixative and not allowed to dry in air
3. Avoid taking the smear when the patient is having a period
4. False-negative smears occur both due to improper technique and laboratory reporting error

## THE TARGET PAYMENT SYSTEM FOR CERVICAL CYTOLOGY

1. There are two target levels – 80% and 50%
2. The lower target level will have been reached if 50% of the eligible women on a GP's list who are aged 25 – 64 years (20 – 60 in Scotland) have had an adequate cervical smear taken during the 5.5 years preceding the claim. Note that only adequate smears will count – if a smear has been taken that is inadequate, it will not count towards your target level
3. Women who have had a hysterectomy involving the complete removal of the cervix will be excluded from the target population. GPs must ensure therefore that these women are notified to the Health Authority
4. The size of the payment will depend on three factors:
   (i) The target level achieved – the ratio of payment is to be 3:1 in favour of the higher 80% target
   (ii) The number of women aged 25 – 64 (20 – 60 in Scotland) on the GP's list – the more women eligible the higher the possible payment
   (iii) The percentage of smears taken in the GP's surgery (i.e. by the GP or practice nurse) as opposed to other sources (i.e. Health Authorities, Family Planning Clinics, etc.)

### REFERENCE

McPherson A 1985 Cervical screening: a practical guide. Oxford University Press. Report of the British Medical Association 1986 Cervical cancer and screening in Great Britain.

# Contraception

## ASSESSMENT OF A PATIENT STARTING THE COMBINED PILL FOR THE FIRST TIME

1. GP should take a history to assess the risk factors and contraindications. Particularly note age, past medical history, cardiac disease, diabetes, hypertension, epilepsy, jaundice, deep venous thrombosis (DVT), migraine, family history, smoking, menstrual history, current medication and weight. Enquire about use of contact lenses
2. Helpful to fill in a special oral contraceptive record card to ensure nothing missed
3. As a minimum, at initial consultation check BP and record weight. Test urine for glycosuria, especially if a family history of diabetes
4. A breast examination and/or a pelvic examination may be considered intrusive at the initial consultation with a young girl requesting the pill for the first time
5. Record in the notes rubella status and last cervical smear

## HOW TO TAKE THE COMBINED PILL: WHAT TO TELL THE NEW PATIENT

1. Combined pill can be started on the first day of menstruation, which provides for immediate contraception. The first cycle is shortened and the next pack is started after the 7-day break. Alternatively, if after the first day, start the combined pill on day 5 and use additional contraception for the first 14 days
2. Take the pill at the same time every day for 21 days. During the pill-free days, you will have a withdrawal bleed. If you have a breakthrough bleed do not stop the pill
3. If you forget a pill and the interval is less than 12 h take it, taking the next pill at its usual time. If more than 12 h have elapsed continue the packet but take extra precautions for the next 7 days. If a pill is missed, and there are less than 7 pills in the pack, the next pack should be started without a break

4. With diarrhoea/vomiting or use of antibiotics, continue the packet but follow the rules in 3 above for a missed pill
5. After the above explanation, issue an explanatory booklet and answer any questions or worries the patient may have about the pill, e.g. any side-effects she may have heard of

## CONTRAINDICATIONS TO THE COMBINED PILL

### Absolute
1. Pregnancy
2. Liver disease/impaired liver function
3. Undiagnosed vaginal bleeding
4. Carcinoma of uterus or breast, malignant melanoma and hepatoma
5. Cardiovascular system
   (i) Moderate or severe hypertension
   (ii) History of thromboembolism (deep venous thrombosis, pulmonary embolism, cerebrovascular accident, myocardial infarction, transient ischaemic attack and atrial fibrillation as a predisposing cause)
   (iii) Certain cardiac anomalies
6. History of herpes gestationis
7. Deterioration of otosclerosis during pregnancy
8. Sickle cell anaemia
9. Porphyria
10. Pituitary disease
11. Recent hydatidiform mole
12. Long-term immobilization
13. Four weeks prior to elective major surgery

### Relative
1. Mild hypertension ⎫
2. Hyperlipidaemia   ⎪
3. Age over 35 years ⎬ Risk factors for a thrombosis
4. Obesity           ⎪
5. Smoking           ⎭
6. Diabetes mellitus
7. Migraine
8. Renal disease
9. Epilepsy – if on anticonvulsants, use a higher-dose pill
10. Asthma
11. Depression
12. Oligo- or amenorrhoea
13. Lactation
14. Fibroids
15. Varicose veins (see below)

16. Gall stones
17. Contact lenses

*Notes:*
1. While one relative risk factor may be acceptable two may not – err on the side of caution. Also, different degrees of risk factor, e.g. a diabetic with evidence of arteriopathy would be an absolute contraindication
2. Infective hepatitis only a contraindication when the liver function tests (LFTs) are abnormal – best to wait a full year
3. Varicose veins not contraindications unless a previous thrombosis, recent operation or sclerotherapy, or they are severe. Uncertain whether a history of superficial thrombophlebitis should be regarded as a contraindication

## SIGNIFICANT MAJOR PROBLEMS OF THE COMBINED PILL

1. Cerebral thrombosis
2. Myocardial infarction
3. Pulmonary embolism
4. Deep vein thrombosis
5. Severe hypertension
6. Severe depression
7. Severe migraine
8. Hepatic tumours – but increased risk small
9. Cholestatic jaundice
10. Reduced glucose tolerance
11. Possible effect on carcinoma of the cervix but this may be more a reflection of sexual activity than actual risk. More worrying is a possible increased risk (albeit a very low increased risk) of breast cancer with total duration of use in younger patients (see UK National Care-Control Study Group reference), but at present there seems no reason to change current guidelines. Oral contraceptives do protect against endometrial and ovarian cancer

*Note*: Stop the pill if any of the above, but diabetics may only need adjustment of their therapy. Also stop if pregnant, immobilized or 4 weeks before an operation. Common side-effects of the pill, with suggested remedies, are noted in Table 13

*Drug interactions*
The effectiveness of the combined pill can be reduced by some anticonvulsants, some antibiotics (e.g. amoxycillin, tetracyclines), some tranquillizers and griseofulvin

**Follow-up**
1. If starting the pill, review in 3 months

**Table 13**    Common side-effects and problems

| Side-effect | Suggested remedy |
|---|---|
| Nausea | Try a lower oestrogen dose |
| Depression | Try pyridoxine 50 mg bd |
| Weight gain | Diet |
| Breakthrough bleeding | Common in first or second cycle. May need to increase dose |
| Hypertension | If diastolic BP>90 mmHg on two occasions, stop the pill |
| Acne | Reduce progestogen dose and use a higher oestrogenic pill |

2. Check BP every 6 months
3. Record weight initially
4. Teach breast self-examination early on and check patient's technique
5. Test urine if indicated (FH of diabetes, history of gestational diabetes, large babies, etc.)
6. Discourage smoking
7. Check rubella status
8. Cervical smear every 3 years

## PROGESTOGEN-ONLY PILL

For patients
1. With diabetes mellitus
2. Who are lactating
3. Over 40 years (35 if a smoker)
4. Who develop significant side-effects on the combined pill
Taken at the same time every day, regardless of menstruation. Effective for only about 21 h, hence best taken at night (assuming intercourse at night). Main problem is menstrual irregularity (irregular bleeding, spotting, menorrhagia, etc.)

## POSTCOITAL CONTRACEPTION

Schering have produced a special PC4 pack (Schering PC4). The dose is 2 tablets as soon as possible after intercourse (up to 72 h after), repeated in 12 h.

## THE IUCD

Try and avoid in nullips (risk of pelvic infection and subsequent infertility)

### Contraindications
1. Pregnancy
2. Previous or present pelvic infection (not *Candida* or *Trichomonas*)
3. Previous ectopic pregnancy
4. Uterine neoplasms, including cervical malignancy
5. Abnormality of the uterus or fibroids
6. Women on steroids or immunosuppressives (reduced contraception and risk of infection)
7. Undiagnosed vaginal bleeding
8. Menorrhagia
9. Cardiac lesions with a risk of endocarditis
10. Allergy to copper (for copper devices)

### Fitting
1. Learn the technique at the local Family Planning Clinic
2. Best inserted during or just after menstruation
3. Can be inserted immediately termination or postpartum at the postnatal examination
4. Discuss with the patient common problems (increased menstrual loss and pain after insertion). Explain about feeling for threads, demonstrate the device and advise not to use tampons for the next two periods
5. The newer copper-containing devices need changing every 5 years (e.g. Nova T and Novagard)

### Problems and side-effects
1. Pregnancy—consider the possibility of an ectopic. If can see threads, remove the IUCD
2. Perforation
3. Expulsion – if in doubt ultrasound
4. Pain – for dysmenorrhoea try Ponstan
5. Menorrhagia – may settle. Check the haemoglobin
6. Infection (including actinomycosis). Minor infections may respond to metronidazole and tetracycline but if unresponsive, or other than minor, remove the IUCD

### Follow-up
Check position of the IUCD in 2 months, then yearly

## THE DIAPHRAGM
1. Learn how to fit diaphragms

2. A good method in well-motivated women, in conjunction with spermicide
3. Spermicide available as cream or jelly
4. Check for size post-pregnancy, after a pelvic operation or after a change in weight
5. Check the patient is happy fitting the diaphragm herself, issue an explanatory leaflet and discuss the main points (leave in for at least 6 h after intercourse, etc.)

## OTHER METHODS OF CONTRACEPTION

1. Condom
2. Cervical caps
3. Rhythm method
4. Temperature method      Unreliable compared with
5. Mucus method            other methods
6. Withdrawal

## DEPOT PROGESTOGENS

Intramuscular injection of Depo-Provera every 12 weeks. Irregular bleeding common. Best used as a stop-gap, e.g. after a vasectomy awaiting negative sperm counts

## NORPLANT

A subdermal implant of the progestogen levonorgestrel providing up to 5 years contraception. GPs can be trained to insert. Read data sheet for further details

## STERILIZATION

### Vasectomy
Needs two negative sperm counts with a month between the specimens before can dispense with other precautions

### Laparoscopic sterilization
Immediately effective but involves a general anaesthetic

# Ante- and postnatal care

## PREGNANCY TEST

1. Urine tests rely on detection of HCG in urine
2. Routine tests positive 10–14 days after missed period but newer tests accurate within a day or two of missed period
3. False-positives occur
   (i) After a recent miscarriage
   (ii) With proteinuria
   (iii) Due to gonadotrophins – FSH at the menopause and with infertility drugs
4. False-negatives occur
   (i) If tested too early or too late (16–18 weeks)
   (ii) If not an early morning specimen
   (iii) If test performed incorrectly

Contamination and drugs (e.g. phenothiazines) may interfere with testing. Gestation sac detected by scan at 6 weeks. By 8 weeks should be able to detect enlargement of uterus vaginally. Also a sensitive blood test for β-HCG now available

## BOOKING PROCEDURE

1. History
   (i) Menstrual, LMP, expected date of delivery (EDD) = 9 months + 7 days from the first day of last menstrual period
   (ii) Previous obstetric and gynaecological history
   (iii) Marital and social history
   (iv) Family history (twins, diabetes, etc.)
2. Physical parameters
   (i) Height and shoe size
   (ii) Weight
   (iii) Physical examination if appropriate
3. Antenatal parameters as per cooperation card (urine, weight, BP, etc.)
4. Advice about antenatal care, breastfeeding, smoking, alcohol, taking of iron supplements and self medication

*Note*: otherwise healthy women do not need routine iron supplements. Reserve these for those at risk of anaemia. More important is the evidence that folic acid supplement, may help prevent neural tube defects. All women should be advised to take 0.4 mg daily of folate prior to conception and in the first 12 weeks of pregnancy (5 mg if they have already had an affected baby)
  5. Tests
      (i)  Blood group and rhesus antibodies
     (ii)  VDRL or other test for syphilis
    (iii)  Test for immunity to rubella
     (iv)  AFP at 16–18 weeks
      (v)  Scan if unsure dates, large for dates, etc.
     (vi)  MSU – often included
    (vii)  Check on cervical cytology status

## CRITERIA FOR BOOKING IN A GP RATHER THAN A CONSULTANT UNIT

  1. Nulliparae over 5 ft in height, aged between 20 and 30 years
  2. Second or third pregnancies, providing patient under 35 years
  3. No previous abnormality in the medical (e.g. diabetes), obstetric (e.g. previous postpartum haemorrhage, previous manual removal of placenta, caesarean section, etc.) or gynaecological history
  4. No rhesus antibodies
  5. No previous psychiatric problems

Once booked in a GP unit, refer to a consultant unit if any problems or anticipated problems arise (twins diagnosed, breech presentation in later pregnancy, pre-eclampsia, etc.)

## ROUTINE ANTENATAL CARE

Every 4 weeks to 28 weeks
Every 2 weeks from 28 to 36 weeks
Weekly from 36 weeks

## USEFUL NOTES ON PARAMETERS AND TESTS IN PREGNANCY

### Size
  1. Palpable abdominally at 12 weeks
  2. Usually below umbilicus at 20 weeks but above it at 24 weeks
  3. Palpation not as accurate as measuring height of fundus from the symphysis pubis in centimetres

### Fetal movements
  1. Usually felt between 16 and 18 weeks in multips, 18 and 20 weeks in primigravidae

2. Many units now use 'kick charts' as a guide to fetal progress, decreasing movements being an indication for fetal monitoring, notably using the cardiotocograph (CTG)

**Presenting part**
As a general rule, if not cephalic by 34 weeks, a consultant opinion should be sought. Beware the 'high head at term' (? disproportion, placenta praevia, etc.)

**Blood pressure**
1. Mild hypertension $\geqslant \frac{140}{90}$ or $> \frac{30}{20}$ mmHg increase from the booking BP
2. Severe hypertension $\geqslant \frac{160}{100}$ mmHg
3. Hypertension can be pre-existing or pregnancy induced
4. Mild pre-eclampsia would have a BP $\geqslant \frac{140}{90}$ mmHg (but $< \frac{160}{100}$ mmHg). Best referred to hospital at this stage and if BP rises above $\frac{140}{90}$ mmHG or proteinuria develops referral is mandatory

*Three key points*
(i) Proteinuria (in absence of UTI) is a danger signal
(ii) Trigger criteria in assessment of BP is $\frac{150}{90}$ or $> \frac{30}{20}$ mmHg over booking or prepregnancy level
(iii) Slight oedema is the rule rather than the exception but watch for sudden weight gain

**Urine**
1. Proteinuria: if not due to pre-eclampsia may be due to asymptomatic UTI – take an MSU
2. Glycosuria: may be low renal threshold but if on two occasions or once in early pregnancy (< 16 weeks) it is advisable to do a GTT (glucose tolerance test), usually at 32 weeks, to detect a gestational diabetes

**Weight**
1. Great variation in weight gain – usually 10–14 kg
2. In latter half of pregnancy excess weight gain (1 kg or more a week) may be a sign of developing pre-eclampsia
3. Static weight or weight loss may mean intrauterine growth retardation

**Other tests in pregnancy**
1. Haemoglobin – aim to keep above 10 g/dl

2. If rhesus-negative a blood test(s) will be needed for antibodies later in pregnancy
3. Oestriols are increasingly used to monitor the latter few weeks of pregnancy
4. AFP is taken at 16–18 weeks as a screen for neural tube defects. Refer if raised, after taking a repeat sample. May of course have been taken at wrong gestation (confirm dates) or be a twin pregnancy

**Antepartum haemorrhage (bleeding after 28 weeks)**
Treat seriously – refer *all* cases and *never* do a vaginal examination (VE) prior to referral

## TREATMENT OF SOME COMMON PROBLEMS IN PREGNANCY

1. Nausea and vomiting – usually resolves about 14–16 weeks. If severe, exclude infection. Promethazine (Avomine) if severe and needs medication
2. Heartburn – antacids safe in second and third trimester, e.g. Mucaine or Gaviscon
3. Constipation – best treatment is to increase fibre intake
4. Infection – UTI and asymptomatic bacteriuria must be treated (risk of pyelonephritis). Penicillins are safe and nitrofurantoin a second choice for UTI. Avoid tetracyclines and co-trimoxazole and metronidazole in first trimester
5. Candidiasis – Canesten pessaries are safe
6. Haemorrhoids – high-fibre diet and Anusol ointment
7. Varicose veins – support tights and avoid excess standing

## THE POSTNATAL PERIOD

GPs are paid a fee for up to five postnatal visits (although these can be carried out by the midwife) and the postnatal examination between 6 and 12 weeks.
  Postnatal problems include:
1. Pyrexia (> 38°) – consider genital tract infection, UTI, breast and chest infections. Also remember DVT
2. Secondary postpartum haemorrhage (PPH) – blood loss more than 24 h after confinement. Many settle. Exclude infection. If more than slight or uterus enlarged and non-involuting (i.e. ? retained products) refer
3. Psychiatric problems – 'baby blues' common on third and fourth day but can get a true psychosis. Do not underestimate a psychosis or a true postnatal depression – there is a real risk to mother and baby. Refer for a psychiatric opinion
4. DVT – Remember! Older patients, obese patients and after

caesarean, especially at risk. Pulmonary embolism commonest cause of death in puerperium

## THE POSTNATAL EXAMINATION

Routine postnatal usually involves seven areas for the GP:
1. Uterus – never returns to size of nullip. By 10 days has usually returned to pelvis. Also check episiotomy site
2. Breasts – encourage breastfeeding
3. Check on rubella and cervical cytology status. Organize as appropriate
4. Discuss any problems of the pregnancy, e.g. check BP of those who were hypertensive, consider referral for IVP if pyelonephritis of pregnancy, etc.
5. Contraception. An IUCD may be fitted postnatally, the mini-pill prescribed for those breastfeeding or the combined pill for those not
6. The baby. A good time to mention immunization, check on registration of baby and ask about any worries
7. Ensure claim forms for maternity work and contraception are submitted to the FPC

## DRUGS AND BREASTFEEDING

Common drugs to avoid include:

Aminophylline
β-blockers
Benzodiazepines in higher doses
Carbimazole

Phenothiazine derivatives
Salicylates
Tetracyclines
Corticosteroids in higher dose (> 10 mg/day)

Co-trimoxazole
Ergot/ergotamine preparations
Oral hypoglycaemics
Nalidixic acid

Thyroxine
Warfarin
Indomethacin

*Note*: Remember to avoid oestrogen-containing contraceptives, i.e. the combined pill

Common drugs thought to be reasonably safe for breastfeeding mothers are:

Antacids
Antihistamines
Chlormethiazole
Cimetidine
Codeine
Digoxin
Heparin
Methyldopa

Naproxen
Nitrazepam
Paracetamol
Penicillins
Trimethoprim
Erythromycin
Insulin

# Orthopaedics and joints

**BACKACHE**

**Diagnosis**

Two processes here:

1. Is it mechanical backache or is there some underlying pathology? Remember:
   - (i) The older patient with possibilities of osteoarthrosis, osteoporosis, Paget's disease and malignant deposits in the spine. In the elderly an X-ray may be worthwhile
   - (ii) The young patient with low back pain and morning stiffness who may have ankylosing spondylitis
   - (iii) Referred pain – renal or gynaecological
   - (iv) Infection
   - (v) Depression – can present as backache

   Mechanical backache is likely to be episodic, related to posture, worse on movement and relieved by rest. Back pain without these features, in the young (< 20 years), in the elderly, that is progressive or continuous, or associated with systemic symptoms demands fuller investigation

2. If the pain is mechanical is it due to a prolapsed intervertebral disc? Practically this means, are there symptoms of nerve root compression?

**Examination**

1. Observe the curvature, feel where the tenderness is and test movement
2. Important part is the testing of straight leg raising (SLR) and the femoral stretch test (knee flexion when prone), the latter to detect higher (L 3/4) root pressure
3. A motor and sensory examination together with testing the reflexes is not likely to be a feature of the examination unless a disc prolapse is suspected
4. Much can be learnt from patient's demeanour and posture and by simple enquiry (? sciatica, ? recent injury, ? occupation, etc.)

5. The rare central disc prolapse presents with urinary symptoms and severe weakness of the legs peripherally and requires an immediate referral for emergency surgery

**Investigation**
1. A plain X-ray is of limited value in mechanical backache/disc prolapse although a 'normal' X-ray does have its reassuring function in the occasional patient
2. For the non-mechanical group a plain X-ray, full-blood count and ESR is advisable, including a prostate-specific antigen for the elderly male and an alkaline phosphatase for the older patient of either sex. Indeed it might be prudent to do a rectal examination, listen to the chest and feel the breasts of any elderly patient with undiagnosed back pain
3. Under 20s and over 60s should be investigated

**Notes on management**
1. In general practice at least 80% recover in 4 weeks
2. For simple 'ligamentous' backache, give simple advice on lifting, analgesia and perhaps a few days off work
3. For disc prolapse with nerve root compression, the patient should have a *minimum* of 3 weeks' bed rest with regular analgesia. Diazepam is a good muscle relaxant and should be used to supplement the analgesia. Check on patient's progress. If, in spite of this regime, strictly adhered to, there is deterioration, worsening of SLR, developing neurological signs, etc., then refer to hospital for further assessment. Occasionally referral for the 3 weeks' bed rest may have to be considered because the home environment is unsuitable
4. Also refer suspected disease rather than mechanical back pain
5. Remember central disc prolapse as an emergency referral – beware of urinary symptoms
6. Manipulation may be useful for some minor mechanical backaches (not prolapsed discs) and it is worth watching a GP experienced with manipulation

**Newer techniques**
Injection techniques are increasingly being used and GPs should be aware of their value, especially in helping the sufferer from a prolapsed disc. Paravertebral nerve blocks and epidural injections are now in common use and discolysis (injecting a herniated disc with the enzyme chymopapain) may save an operation. For the very few laminectomy is still the only answer.

**CERVICAL SPONDYLOSIS**
1. Common in middle to later adult life

2. Remissions and relapses
3. Commonest symptoms are pain in the neck or occiput radiating into shoulder of upper arms
4. Restriction of neck movement in a collar helps
5. Refer for surgery if symptoms of cervical cord compression or vertebrobasilar ischaemia exacerbated by moving the neck – surgery very rarely needed

## LIMP IN A CHILD

1. Refer for full evaluation
2. Perthes' presents usually about age 4–10 years, slipped upper femoral epiphysis over the age of 10 years

## THE PAINFUL KNEE

Typically there are three groups of patients:
1. Younger age group with knee pain but no history of trauma. Consider:
    (i) Referred pain from hip (e.g. Perthes' 4–10 years, slipped epiphysis > 10 years)
    (ii) Osgood-Schlatter's disease – in adolescents with pain over tibial tubercle. Advise no sport for at least 3 months. A benign condition
    (iii) Chondromalacia patellae – especially young females. Pain in patella ± swelling, especially when climbing stairs. Avoid sport except swimming. If symptoms severe and persistent may need patellectomy
2. Young or middle-aged adults with an injury. Assess the degree of injury:
    (i) The history – including any rotation or twist
    (ii) Degree of swelling. Is there any blood in the knee?
    (iii) Pain and limitation of movements
    (iv) Ability of patient to walk
Object is to detect complete rupture of ligaments, complete tears of the meniscus, fractures or dislocations, i.e. conditions requiring possible operative intervention

As a general rule refer for hospital assessment:
    (i) If there was a definite crack or click during the injury
    (ii) If there is 'locking', i.e. patient cannot fully extend the knee
    (iii) Severe knee injury, especially if a tense haemarthrosis requires tapping
    (iv) Instability – the knee 'gives way'
If none of those apply prescribe NSAIDs and bandage, reviewing in a few days. If there is then failure of extension of the knee or it 'gives way', refer

3. Pain in the middle-aged to elderly patient with no injury. Consider gout, osteoarthritis and rheumatoid arthritis. *Note*: At any age remember a septic arthritis

## THE SPRAINED ANKLE

Primary decision is to exclude a fracture or complete tear of the lateral ligament. X-ray severe injuries, those with tenderness other than the ligament area and where there is instability or undue movement at the joint. If no fracture or complete tear is suspected the treatment of a sprained ankle is:
1. In the acute phase ice, ultrasound (if available) and elevation
2. Analgesia, e.g. naproxen
3. Strapping in the form of a 'U-stirrup', i.e. a U-stirrup of orthopaedic felt to give support and then an Elastoplast dressing round the ankle and foot, and up the calf, to end at the tibial tubercle. Practice nurse can aid the GP by learning this technique

### Practical notes
1. Severe sprains should be treated in plaster of Paris
2. May be that even if lateral ligament has been completely torn conservative treatment in plaster of Paris can be used rather than immediate surgical repair (see Lightowler 1984)

## THE PAINFUL SHOULDER

The acutely painful shoulder of the rotator cuff variety (causing a painful arc syndrome) often responds to an injection of steroid and lignocaine (e.g. Depo-Medrone with Lidocaine) into the subacromial bursa (see Fig. 2)

Frozen shoulders may respond to an intra-articular injection of steroid (e.g. Depo-Medrone, Lederspan). There are various approaches to the shoulder joint – I prefer the posterior approach. The techniques can only be learnt by practical example.

*Note*: Polymyalgia rheumatica can present as pain and stiffness of the shoulders – take a good history

## RHEUMATOID ARTHRITIS

1. Management multidisciplinary – district nurse, occupational therapist, home helps, etc.
2. GPs role to maintain morale, detect complications (anaemia, eye problems, etc.) and monitor drug therapy
3. Drug ladder for rheumatoid arthritis:

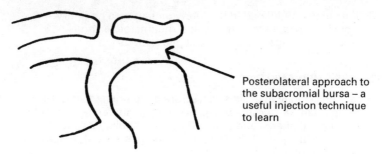

Posterolateral approach to
the subacromial bursa – a
useful injection technique
to learn

**Fig. 2**

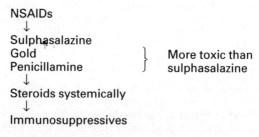

NSAIDs
↓
Sulphasalazine
Gold            } More toxic than
Penicillamine  } sulphasalazine
↓
Steroids systemically
↓
Immunosuppressives

4. More severe cases managed by GP and hospital – a shared care
   system
5. Typical history of joint pains and morning stiffness warrants a
   rheumatoid factor and ESR. Note that a negative rheumatoid
   factor does not exclude rheumatoid arthritis – may be positive
   in only 70% of cases
6. Remember polymyalgia rheumatica – pain and stiffness in
   shoulders and arms, high ESR, negative rheumatoid factor.
   Associated with temporal arteritis

**EC sulphasalazine (Salazopyrin EN tablets)**
1. Used for treatment of rheumatoid arthritis unresponsive to the
   NSAIDs
2. Relatively rapid onset of action: 4–8 weeks
3. Contraindications are sensitivity to sulphonamides or
   salicylates
4. Side-effects include headache, rash, raised temperature,
   hypersensitivity reactions (Stevens-Johnson syndrome,
   photosensitivity reactions, skin eruptions), agranulocytosis,
   CNS reactions, proteinuria and hepatitis
5. Follow-up: FBC + platelets + LFTs monthly for 3 months and
   test urine

## GOUT

1. Remember it may be secondary to disease (e.g. myeloproliferative disorders) or diuretics
2. Many people have asymptomatic hyperuricaemia but do not develop gout
3. For acute attacks try diclofenac (Voltarol) – starting with an injection. Avoid if history of indigestion/peptic ulcer or sensitivity to anti-inflammatory agents
4. For prevention maintenance dose of allopurinol is 200–600 mg/day but remember it can itself precipitate gout. Never start at the time of an attack – wait until settled and then introduce under cover of anti-inflammatory, starting at 100 mg daily and increasing over 3 weeks. Monitor uric acid levels

**Table 14**    Some common orthopaedic problems

|  | Description | Treatment |
|---|---|---|
| 1. Ganglion | Cystic lump common on the dorsum of hand or wrist | Recurrence common. Best treatment is surgical excision |
| 2. Bunion | Pain and inflammation over the first metatarsal head | (i) Use of wide shoes with soft padding to protect the bunion<br>(ii) Surgery, e.g. a Keller's operation |
| 3. Plantar fascilitis | Usually in middle-aged adults a pain and tenderness beneath the calcaneum. Can be associated, especially in younger patients, with Reiter's syndrome and other arthropathies | (i) A pad to relieve pressure on the point<br>(ii) Injection of hydrocortisone worth a try |
| 4. Tennis elbow | Pain and tenderness over the lateral epicondyle of the humerus at the site of the origin of the forearm extensor muscles. X-rays not useful | Try an injection of steroid plus 1% lignocaine into the tender site, injecting deep and down to the bone. If no improvement in 2–3 weeks, try again. Warn patient pain is exacerbated by the injection. Resistant tennis elbow may need surgery |

# Surgery

## HAEMORRHOIDS

1. Advise on a high-fibre diet
2. Suppositories or ointments, e.g. Anusol but beware of sensitivity reactions and subsequent pruritus and hence use for short periods only – especially steroid-containing ointments, which can cause atrophy of the perianal skin
3. Large or persistent haemorrhoids need injection/banding or haemorrhoidectomy

*Note:* If a patient presents with rectal bleeding it is mandatory to take a proper history and perform a digital rectal examination and proctoscopy. Not practical in general practice to refer every patient with piles or an anal tear for a sigmoidoscopy to exclude a coexisting carcinoma higher up but refer those with rectal bleeding

1. If over 40 years
2. If there is a change in bowel habit
3. If the blood is mixed with mucus
4. If there is associated abdominal pain
5. If the blood is dark and mixed with the stool rather than fresh
6. If there is a history (or family history) of polyps
7. If there is recurrent or persistent bleeding
8. If there is severe bleeding

Rectal bleeding with no obvious cause despite rectal examination, i.e. not due to piles, tears, etc., must obviously be referred for full investigation, including sigmoidoscopy

## A LUMP IN THE BREAST

One in 12 British women develops breast cancer

### History
Ask the patient:

1. Length of history – when and how first noticed?
2. Is it getting bigger?

3. Associated symptoms, i.e. pain, discharge, retraction or bleeding
4. Relation of symptoms to periods
5. Past history or family history of breast problems
6. Medication (the pill, hormone replacement therapy)

**Examination**
1. Examine the four quadrants of both breasts, the axillae and the supraclavicular fossae
2. If a lump is found, is it mobile or fixed to skin, hard or soft and cystic, regular or irregular?

**Management**
1. Refer all discrete lumps
2. If a lumpy breast but no discrete lumps as such, recheck after a period
3. Some aspirate cystic lumps in young women, refer if the fluid is bloodstained or there is a remaining lump after aspiration or the lump recurs

**UK National Breast Screening Programme**
1. The Health Insurance Plan study in New York (Shapiro et al 1977) showed that clinical examination combined with mammography can detect carcinomas at a stage early enough to significantly reduce mortality (in the over 50s studied). Recent studies in Sweden and the UK breast screening trial have confirmed the value of mammography in reducing breast cancer mortality in the over 50s
2. Following the recommendations of the Forrest Report in 1986, a National Breast Screening Programme has now been introduced in the UK. The guidelines are:
    (i) To screen women aged 50–64 by single oblique view mammography. Fifty was chosen as it is from this age that mammography has been shown to reduce mortality significantly (breast cancer rising dramatically with age)
    (ii) The screening interval between mammograms is to be 3 years
    (iii) GPs will receive a 'prior notification list' so that they can check patients are still on the list, live at the quoted address and have no specific reason why they shouldn't be screened. The computerized call invitations are based on this corrected list
    (iv) Each locality will have its own specific protocols based on the national guidelines. It is important that GPs become acquainted with the running of their local system

## A VENOUS LEG ULCER

### Diagnosis
Differentiate from
1. Arterial ulcers (check peripheral pulses)
2. Diabetic ulcers (check urine for sugar)
3. Traumatic ulcers
4. Vasculitic ulcers of an autoimmune condition

### Management
1. Varicose veins themselves treated by elastic support stockings, injection and stripping
2. Mainstay of treatment is cleansing, compression and elevation
   (i) Clean ulcer with saline or potassium permanganate. Do not use topical antibiotics or other ointments (danger of sensitization). Varicose eczema responds to 1% hydrocortisone but do not use steroids near an ulcer edge
   (ii) Apply a zinc paste bandage (e.g. Viscopaste) from toes to the knees and over this apply a firm crepe bandage (an Elastocrepe firmly applied provides good compression)
   (iii) Patient can walk short distances but to avoid prolonged standing and to elevate the leg at rest and at night
3. Larger infected ulcers may need a course of amoxycillin plus metronidazole
4. Treat associated problems, i.e. the varicose veins, obesity, congestive cardiac failure, diabetes, anaemia. Ensure adequate nutrition
5. If not healing, consider referral for intensive hospital treatment and even skin grafting. An ulcer failing to heal in 6 months or with a rolled edge may be a carcinoma
6. To prevent recurrence once healed, remember elastic support stockings

## PRACTICAL NOTES ON DIAGNOSING THE CAUSE OF ACUTE ABDOMINAL PAIN

### Three golden rules:
1. Take time in eliciting a full history before the examination. Do not skip the conventional site, character, radiation, etc., and remember to ask the date of the last menstrual period in a female patient (? ectopic)
2. Assume the worst until proved otherwise, i.e. start by thinking of appendicitis, perforated peptic ulcer, intestinal obstruction and exclude rather than assume gastroenteritis and be proved wrong. If in doubt review in 2 h but if suspicion sufficiently aroused admit. Err on the side of caution
3. Examine carefully and methodically, thus:

   (i)  How 'ill' or in pain is the patient – some diagnoses speak for themselves, e.g. rolling around in agony with renal colic

  (ii)  Take the temperature – unusual to be appendicitis without a pyrexia

 (iii)  With regard to the abdominal examination do not forget the hernial orifices (? strangulated hernia) and the testes (? torsion)

 (iv)  Remember to perform a rectal examination

  (v)  Test the urine as appropriate

**Three general rules:**

1. As a general rule abdominal pain lasting longer than 6 h is likely to require hospital admission
2. Avoid antibiotics and analgesics, which may mask the diagnosis unless obvious, e.g. renal colic
3. Symptoms and signs can be classed into two groups:
   - (i) Generally less serious
     - Diarrhoea
     - Afebrile patient
     - Normal pulse
     - Soft abdomen
     - Past history of similar episodes
     - Recent respiratory infection or dietary indiscretion
   - (ii) Potentially more serious
     - Vomiting
     - Febrile patient
     - Tachycardia
     - Tenderness, rigidity
     - Severe pain, worsening pain or pain lasting longer than 6 h

However, beware pelvic appendicitis, which may cause diarrhoea or urinary symptoms and may only be detectable on rectal examination

*Note*: Even if confident the cause of the abdominal pain is innocent and you are not revisiting, explain to the patient or relatives what to expect and when to call for a revisit if the patient's condition fails to improve

## ENDOSCOPY VERSUS BARIUM MEAL IN THE INVESTIGATION OF DYSPEPSIA

1. Patients over the age of 40 years presenting with dyspepsia for the first time should be referred for endoscopy – there is a 1 in 50 chance they will have a gastric carcinoma. Allum et al (1986) conducted a study where GPs referred all those over 40 years

presenting with dyspepsia for endoscopy – 15 out of 683 had gastric cancer and 79 had precancerous histological changes
2. Postendoscopy if a duodenal ulcer/hiatus hernia has been found it is reasonable to treat recurrences with antacids/$H_2$ antagonists or consider *Helicobacter pylori* eradication therapy (see below)
3. Do not use $H_2$ antagonists as first-line treatment in dyspeptic patients over 40 years – they can mask the symptoms of a carcinoma

## TREATMENT OF DUODENAL ULCER

Cimetidine 400 mg bd or 800 mg nocte, ranitidine 150 mg bd or 300 mg nocte or omeprazole 20 mg daily for 4 weeks. Surgery rarely needed except for the few resistant to treatment, bleeding or perforation

*Helicobacter pylori eradication*
Over 80% of patients with treated duodenal ulcers relapse within a year. This can be reduced to 10% by eradicating *H. pylori* and there is now an excellent case for eradicating *H. pylori* in patients with duodenal ulcers. Triple therapy with bismuth (De-Nol), metronidazole and amoxycillin is less acceptable to patients than the alternative — omeprazole 20 mg b.d. and amoxycillin 1 g b.d., both for 14 days

## MINOR SURGERY IN GENERAL PRACTICE

1. GPs, under the 1990 Contract, receive a fee for minor surgery, providing they are on their Health Authority's Minor Surgery List. The first step to qualifying for payment is therefore to convince the Health Authority you have the training/experience/equipment to merit inclusion in the Minor Surgery List
2. The payment system works as follows:
   (i) A GP will be able to claim for three sessional payments in any one quarter
   (ii) Each session will consist of at least five surgical procedures. The procedures can be carried out together in one clinic session or they can be performed on separate occasions during the quarter
   (iii) A GP can also perform minor surgery on patients on the list of his partners and in this case will be able to claim more sessional payments (up to three times the number of partners per quarter)
3. The surgical procedures which will count towards a session are:

- Certain injections (intra-articular, periarticular, injections for varicose veins and haemorrhoids)
- Aspirations of joints, cysts, bursae and hydroceles
- Incisions of abscesses, cysts and thrombosed piles
- Excisions of sebaceous cysts, lipomas, skin lesions and warts
- Removal of toenails (partial and complete)
- Curetting, cautery or cryocautery of warts, verrucae and other skin lesions
- Removal of foreign bodies
- Nasal cautery

# Practice management

TERMS OF SERVICE FOR GPs UNDER THE NEW 1990 CONTRACT

**Reference:** Terms of Service for Doctors and General Practice. Department of Health 1989

The main points are listed below:

1. A GP is required to offer patients general medical services including referral as appropriate, immunizations, advice on general health (especially diet, exercise, smoking, alcohol and the misuse of drugs) and consultations/examinations to reduce the risk of disease or injury
2. A GP is remunerated for providing child health surveillance services, providing he or she qualifies for the Child Health Surveillance List (*see* Paediatrics chapter). Similarly a GP is remunerated for providing minor surgery services providing he qualifies for the Minor Surgery List (*see* Surgery chapter)
3. A GP should be available
   - in 42 weeks out of 52 weeks
   - for 26 hours in any such week
   - for 5 days in any such week

There is a clause allowing certain doctors (e.g. those heavily involved in teaching/training) to be available on only 4 days a week. The 26 hours will include visiting but not 'on call' time

4. A GP is required to offer (in writing) all newly registered patients (except children under 5) a health promotion consultation within 28 days of accepting them onto the list. This New Registration Check includes
   (i) Taking a medical history of
      a. Current state of health
      b. Medication and allergies
      c. Past illnesses/hereditary conditions
      d. Immunization/cervical smear/mammography status
      e. Diet/exercise/smoking/alcohol/misuse of drugs
      f. Social factors – employment, housing and family
   (ii) Measuring and testing

      a. Height, weight and blood pressure
      b. The urine for albumin and glucose

5. For patients aged 75 and over, the GP must invite them in writing to attend for a consultation and offer to make to each patient an annual domiciliary visit to assess their needs (*see* Geriatrics chapter)

6. Every practice must have a *practice leaflet* reviewed annually, and a copy of this leaflet must be made available to the Health Authority. The information that must be included in this leaflet is:

    (i) Name, sex, qualifications, date and place of first registration of the medical practitioners
    (ii) Times the GP is available for consultation
    (iii) Details of the appointment system, including how to obtain an urgent or a non-urgent appointment and how to request a domiciliary visit. Also included must be details of the cover provided when a GP is not personally available
    (iv) Details of the repeat prescription system
    (v) If the GP is a dispensing one, the dispensing arrangements
    (vi) Details of the clinics provided by the GP (frequency, duration, purpose)
    (vii) Numbers and roles of attached staff
    (viii) Details of whether the GP
      a. Provides maternity, contraceptive, child surveillance or minor surgery services
      b. Is single-handed or in partnership
      c. Employs an assistant (in which case the assistant's details should be listed as in (i))
    (ix) The arrangements for receiving patient's comments on the services provided
    (x) The access for disabled patients
    (xi) If a training or teaching practice, the arrangements for drawing this to the attention of patients
    (xii) The geographical boundary of the practice by reference to a map

7. An *annual report* must be provided each year to the Health Authority, containing the following information:

    (i) Details of staff – number, duties, hours worked, qualifications and training
    (ii) Details of premises – variations since the last report and anticipated changes in the forthcoming year
    (iii) Details of patient referrals
      – total number referred as in-patients or out-patients and in each case the speciality referred to must be listed (general surgery, ENT, paediatrics, etc.) and the name of the hospital used. Pathology and X-ray are

included, hence you must also note what tests you
ordered
- total number of cases known where patients have
referred themselves (i.e. largely via Casualty)
(iv) Details of a doctor's other commitments – posts held
(clinical assistants, etc.) and 'a description of all work
undertaken'
(v) Details of arrangements whereby the practice receives
patients' comments on the doctor's provision of services
(vi) Details of the repeat prescription system and whether the
doctor uses a separate formulary or the practice has its
own formulary

## COMPLAINTS PROCEDURES

By 1995 GPs will have to have a practice complaints procedure in
operation. Staff should be trained in handling complaints and a
practice will have to report on its complaints procedures annually
to the Health Authority. If the patient is not satisfied with the in-
house dealing of a complaint, there is to be a stage two procedure
whereby complaints are screened by a panel with a lay majority. If
the complaint is then referred onward there is a stage three system
which could involve disciplinary action by the Health Authority or
referral to the GMC.

## GENERAL PRACTICE FUNDHOLDING

**Reference**: Developing NHS Purchasing and GP Fundholding Dept
of Health 1994.
Fundholding is a system whereby a practice is allocated a fund to
cover its expenditure on hospital services (in-patient treatment,
outpatient treatment, diagnostic tests), prescribing, community
nursing services and practice staff. There are 3 types of
fundholding, from 1996:
1. Standard fundholding, for which the minimum list size to
qualify is 5000 patients
2. Community fundholding for practices with 3000+ patients. This
includes staff, drugs, diagnostic tests and community services
but not hospital treatment
3. Total purchasing, where GPs purchase all local hospital and
community care for their patients
To be considered for a fund practice you must have an adequate
computer system in operation. It is possible for practices to
combine together to hold a fund. The scheme is voluntary – you do
not have to hold a fund

### Pros of fundholding

1. Computer costs – to recognize the additional workload, Health Authorities will reimburse computer costs at a higher level than non-fundholding practices (*see* section on computers)
2. You will be allowed to switch money between the different areas – savings made on prescribing, for example, can be used to employ extra staff, improve the practice premises or purchase medical equipment. Savings cannot, however, be used for personal income
3. Fundholders will have a greater choice over where they send their patients, and what they send them for
4. There will be a management allowance (*see* section on Practice Manager) to help in the management of running a budget

### Cons of fundholding

1. The budget may prove to be too small for your needs, necessitating an investigation by the Health Authority, with all the liaisons and meetings that will entail
2. The practice's workload will increase substantially, not least to fulfil the requirement to provide the Health Authority with monthly and annual accounts. GPs will have to monitor closely (and document in detail) every referral made, investigation ordered, prescription written, etc.
3. There may be difficulties if you saved money from the fund one year (and employed, say, a chiropodist) only to find that the next year you overspent (and perhaps have to dismiss the chiropodist)
4. The introduction of a financial element into the consultation may severely damage the doctor – patient relationship. Patients not referred to hospital (or not prescribed the newest drugs) may wonder rightly or wrongly if the decision has been made on clinical grounds or on grounds of cost

## MEDICAL RECORDS

### Functions

The functions of good medical records include:
1. Improving patient care. Some examples of this might be:
    - (i) More efficient management of chronic conditions and illness, e.g. the control of hypertensives
    - (ii) Making diagnosis clearer, e.g. repeated infections in an elderly person heralding maturity-onset diabetes

    (iii) Improving management decisions, e.g. referral for tonsillectomy when there is a history of recurrent tonsillitis

    (iv) Monitoring drug therapy, e.g. oral contraception follow-up, monitoring anticonvulsant levels, lithium levels, etc.

    (v) Eliminating some clinical errors, especially with regard to drug interactions and drug sensitivities. Any possible dangers in this respect should be clearly documented in the records

2. A means of communication between doctors. Especially in larger group practices, a patient may be seen by different doctors and these doctors need to be aware of the current problems and therapy prescribed for the patient

3. A reminder of previous significant events and illnesses in the patient's life, his or her family history and social circumstances

4. A tool in audit and research. Good records are an essential requirement in any such project

5. A means of increasing practice income. Accurate recordkeeping should make it obvious when a claim form for contraception should be completed, when a cervical smear is due, etc.

6. Their use as medicolegal documents. With the current climate of increasing litigation it is essential that records are well kept

**Improving the records**
In an average practice with records in FP5/6 envelopes, a basic seven-point plan to improve the records is:
1. The continuation cards should be put in chronological order and treasury tagged together
2. Hospital letters and the results of investigations should also be arranged in chronological order and fastened together
3. Discard any useless, duplicated, illegible or irrelevant material
4. Insert a summary card in front of the records, detailing major diagnoses and problems in date order
5. The outside of the records should be colour-coded (see below)
6. Children should have an updated immunization and vaccination card in their records
7. Construct a drug treatment card for each patient

**Colour-coding**
There is now a universal system of coloured tags for major diseases as shown in Table 15

**Table 15**

| Tag colour | What it indicates |
|---|---|
| Blue | Hypertension |
| Brown | Diabetes |
| Yellow | Epilepsy |
| Red | Hypersensitivity, e.g. to drugs |
| Green | Tuberculosis |
| White | Long-term maintenance therapy |
| Black | Attempted suicide |
| Chequered black and white | Measles |

### Recording the consultation

The standard continuation card has three columns

1. The first column is for the date
2. The second column (under the asterisk) has space for only one letter viz:
   A = attendance at the surgery
   V = visit
   C = certificate
3. The third column is for clinical notes

In recording clinical notes be guided by the following rules:

1. Make the diagnosis clear, e.g. by boxing the diagnosis:

   TONSILLITIS

2. For simple consultations use the minimum number of words, e.g. 'Tonsillitis. PenV 20'
3. Always indicate if a patient has been referred and where to
4. For vague, imprecise consultations, e.g. non-specific abdominal pain, include important negatives, e.g. no tenderness, rectal examination normal
5. Always record the treatment, preferably with the dosage and number of tablets prescribed
6. Certificates should also be recorded. Record the diagnosis you have written on the certificate, e.g. 'Certificate 2 weeks: Backache'
7. Be wary of using obscure abbreviations, e.g. SOB, PID but some more common ones are permissible, e.g. URTI, UTI, etc.
8. Certain consultations with medicolegal implications need thorough documentation, e.g. accidents, injuries, child abuse, disputes between doctor and patient, and important advice given over the telephone
9. Remember to record any visits made to the patient

### The SOAP formula

One popular method of recording a consultation is the SOAP method. The letters stand for:

S = Subjective. The patient's symptoms – information given by the patient
O = Objective. The findings on examination and investigation
A = Assessment. The doctor's diagnosis, assessment and opinion of the situation
P = Plan. Basically what was done and what plans there are for the future. This is the place to record préscriptions, certificates, referrals, what the patient was told, what management is required and what follow-up planned
A very simple example would be:
S = Backache in the lumbar spine for 2 weeks
O = Full range of movement, no tenderness, straight leg raising 90°, R = L
A = Ligamentous backache
P = Certificate 2 weeks: backache. Prescription: Naprosyn 250 mg bd 30. Review in 2 weeks

**A4 records**
There are a number of practices using the larger A4-sized records. Their spread has been limited by two major factors – the cost and the storage space needed. With the age of the computer with us, the desire to convert all records to A4 records may recede. The advantages and disadvantages of A4 records are:

*Advantages*
1. Plenty of space for recording consultations
2. Easy layout of databases, problem lists, summary sheets, family histories, flow sheets, questionnaires, management plans, etc.
3. Hospital letters and investigations can be filed unfolded and hence are readily available for rapid assessment
4. Better layout of information provides access so that audit and research is less time-consuming
5. If a report on a patient is required (including insurance medical reports), the necessary information can be culled quickly with a minimum of effort

*Disadvantages*
1. Cost: secretarial time, price of folders and sheets, cost of storage space, etc.
2. Space: takes up more space than the conventional medical records envelope, hence more office space, shelving, etc. needed
3. When a patient moves, his or her records move to the new practice and, since the majority of practices do not use A4 records, this entails extra work making up a new record
4. Some pundits would say that the amount of unnecessary information written in the notes expands to fill the space available!

### The age – sex register

This is a collection of cards, each containing essential statistics about a given patient. Male patients have blue cards and females have pink cards. On each card is detailed the patient's name, age, date of birth, current address and date of entry in the register. The cards are stored alphabetically under the year of birth, i.e. the year, say, 1930 begins with patients born in that year with the surname starting in A and ends with those born in that year with the surname starting in Z. Male cards are filed separately from female cards. This manual system will be replaced by a computerized system in most practices within the next few years.

The uses of an age – sex register are:

1. Increasing practice income by checking:
   (i) On the immunization status of patients in trying to reach your target
   (ii) If women have had a cervical smear or are due one, again to try and reach your target
   (iii) With the Health Authority, that you are being correctly and appropriately paid for the patients on your list
2. Planning for the future:
   (i) A practice with a large elderly population will require different planning policies to one with a high proportion of young mothers
   (ii) By following trends you can predict future increases or decreases in list size and even, if you have tagged the cards, in different areas (or branch surgeries) within the practice
3. Screening programmes:
   (i) For developmental surveillance of children
   (ii) Cervical cytology screening of women
   (iii) Screening for hypertension or coronary artery disease risk factors
   (iv) Screening of the elderly
4. Research:
   The age – sex register provides a base or denominator for any recording and, by judicious use of tagging systems, the register can be used with great versatility to examine a wide range of problems. It provides the researcher with a 'control' patient, i.e. one matched for age and sex with the 'case' patient
5. Health promotion checks:
   The register will help in trying to achieve a good coverage of health promotion data (see below)

### Morbidity registers

Increasingly practices are constructing disease registers, recording all the patients with a certain disease or problem. Practices can thus audit their management of these diseases, special clinics can be set up and research projects facilitated. The 'E' book is a sophisticated example of a morbidity register, where at the end of a consultation or visit a doctor fills in on a sheet a specific code number indicating the illness, problems or disease and these details are eventually collected together in a loose-leaf ledger, subdivided into the various conditions. Disease registers are an obligatory part of our new health promotion programmes.

**Computers**
In the 1990s all general practices will become computerized. There is now an overwhelming case for computerization to cope with the changes outlined in the New Contract and, more specifically, with the prospect of fundholding. The functions of a computer are:
1. Managing a budget
   The fundholding scheme, is an enormous managerial exercise, impossible to achieve without computers to document referrals, investigations, prescribing, staff and practice costs. Similarly general cash flow and monitoring of expenditure will be easier using the computer
2. Preparing annual reports
   Whether a budget-holder or not, we all have to prepare annual reports listing details of staff, referrals, premises, etc.
3. Repeat prescription systems
   Most practices are using computers for this monotonous, repetitive task which is ideally suited for computerization
4. Practice accounts
   Simple and complex accounting procedures should be easily assimilated by the computer
5. An age–sex register
   The computer will fulfil all the functions of an age–sex register listed above, only with greater speed of retrieval of information. The other obvious advantage is that it will be able to print all the letters inviting patients to attend for their health checks
6. Recall systems
   The Health Authority's computerized recall system will cover the immunizations and smears and similarly we will receive help with the paediatric surveillance. The system of recall for health promotion checks and for screening the elderly is, however, likely to be an area of concern for the practice computer
7. Disease registers
   A computer is ideally suited to replace the various forms of morbidity register
8. Dispensing
   Large dispensing practices will wish to control their stock using a computerized system

9. Information
   The computers of the future may be of great use in everyday practice as a source of information on various topics. A good example would be drug interactions i.e. you may be able to type in a patient's medication and the computer would detail if a new drug would in any way interact or produce unwanted side-effects
10. Health promotion data
   A key area for computers is the gathering of health promotion data. Any patient attending a consultation can be checked against their computer record for any missing information (e.g. BP, smoking habit) required. The computer can then generate statistics on the practice's coverage of its population in terms of blood pressure recording, recording of smoking habits, etc.

## Costs of computerization
There are two – the cost of starting up and maintenance costs. Health Authorities have discretion on reimbursing costs. Up to 50% of the maintenance, purchase, leasing and upgrading costs can be claimed by non-fundholders. Fundholders can claim up to 75% of their hardware costs and all their maintenance and fundholding software costs.

## THE HEALTH CARE TEAM
The primary health care team includes:
1. The GP(s)
2. The practice ancillary staff – practice manager, secretary and reception staff
3. The practice nurse(s)
4. The district nurse(s)
5. The midwife or midwives
6. The health visitor(s)
7. The social worker(s)
8. Many other professionals (dietitians, physiotherapists, marriage guidance counsellors, etc.) may be attached to a given practice in addition to this basic team

## The practice manager
The responsibilities of the practice manager are:
1. The practice: maintaining its overall efficiency
2. Ancillary staff
   (i) Involvement with appointment and dismissal
   (ii) Training
   (iii) Staff contracts

   (iv) Rotas and holidays

   (v) Personal problems of the staff; maintaining a happy atmosphere

3. Finance (including ? managing a practice budget)

   (i) Monitoring (and maximizing) income from the Health Authority, outside appointments, maternity work, smears, vaccinations, contraceptive work, etc., recall schemes and patient registration (including new registration checks)

   (ii) Monitoring all expenditure

   (iii) National Insurance payments, payment of staff and any outside help

   (iv) Control of the petty cash

   (v) Liaison with the accountants

   (vi) Fundholding

   If a practice becomes a fundholding practice considerably more work will be involved in monitoring the cash flow, contracts with hospitals, prescribing and staff costs. Detailed reports to the Health Authority will have to be provided on a monthly and annual basis

   Management allowances can be claimed from the Health Authority to help here. There will be a management fee to cover costs in the preparatory year prior to taking on a fund (budget) and, once you have become a fundholder, there will be an annual management allowance

4. Premises: ensuring they are kept tidy and in good repair; liaison with cleaners, carpenters, decorators, plumbers, etc.

5. Records: keeping an eye on the records, age–sex register, etc. The inevitable computer will appear here!

6. Doctors

   (i) Ensuring that the practice is developing towards its goals

   (ii) Advising the doctors on financial, staff and legal matters relating to employment law and premises

   (iii) Reporting problems to the doctors and implementing policy decisions

7. Stock control: ordering stationery, forms, equipment, pathology bottles, etc.

8. Dispensing: in dispensing practices, controlling the stock of drugs and the prescriptions dispensed

9. Planning: monitoring the systems for appointments, visiting and repeat prescriptions to cope with expected, or unexpected, changes; collecting statistics on appointments, visits, list sizes, etc., to advise the doctors on planning for the future; preparing practice leaflets and annual reports; monitoring the health promotion activities

10. Overseeing the complaints procedure

**The reception staff**
The duties of the reception staff include:
1. Manning the reception desk: making appointments, accepting new patients, providing information about the practice, booking antenatal and any other clinics, giving out completed prescriptions, collecting fees for various certificates, advising on immunization requirements, etc.
2. Telephone duties: answering the telephone, taking messages, ordering ambulances, etc.
3. The premises: keeping them tidy, keeping the doctors supplied with forms and stationery, dealing with problems in the waiting room (from a lost purse to a screaming infant!)
4. Records. Filing and retrieving the records for the doctors, extracting information as required, updating the records; one person may be delegated to look after the age – sex register. Computer skills are invaluable
5. The post. Opening, filing and passing on to the doctors any relevant post
6. Repeat prescriptions. Administering the practice repeat prescription system
7. Paperwork. Helping fill in some of the numerous forms, e.g. for vaccinations. It is essential, to avoid lost income, that all understand what is claimable
8. Flexibility. Responding to new work, emergencies or patients' problems as appropriate (e.g. helping with the typing if the secretary is ill, or delivering a prescription to an elderly patient)

**The district nurse**
The work of this vital member of the team includes:

*In the treatment room*
1. Dressings, including managing minor accidents and injuries, e.g. bandaging a sprained ankle
2. Venepuncture
3. Injections, e.g. hydroxocobalamin, Modecate
4. Immunizations, including tetanus, typhoid, cholera, flu
5. Suture removal
6. General management of wounds, leg ulcers and burns, including taking swabs
7. Ear syringing
8. Changing pessaries
9. Urine testing
10. Recording weight and blood pressure
11. Assisting with minor surgical procedures, e.g. helping the doctor remove a sebaceous cyst
12. ECG and peak flow recordings
13. May help with screening programmes

In some practices, district nurses may also help in the follow-up of
diabetics, supervise those on diets, and advise and counsel patients
on a wide range of health problems

*At the patient's home*
1. General nursing procedures (dressings, removing sutures,
   injections, venepuncture, giving enemas, recording
   temperature, pulse and blood pressure)
2. Help with managing the elderly and disabled at home, e.g.
   managing catheters, providing ripple beds and incontinence
   pads, assessing nursing requirements, turning bed-ridden
   patients, organizing and suggesting outside help (home
   helps, meals-on-wheels, etc.), help with the provision of
   walking aids, general mobilization of support in the
   community
3. Terminal care
4. Monitoring at-risk patients, especially the elderly
5. Liaison with the night nursing services (crucial in managing a
   patient at home)
6. Liaison with auxiliary nurses, who may help with bathing,
   collecting prescriptions and an awful lot more!
7. Advice on health care in general
8. Knowledge of all the available local support and services, so
   that more help can be given to a specific patient
9. Social support: the nurse becomes a trusted personal and
   family friend

**The practice nurse**
With the advent of the New Contract, practice nurses have become
a key member of the health care team. New and important areas of
possible responsibility are:
1. Health promotion activities (see below)
2. New registration checks
3. Developing and participating in the practice's programme for
   asthma and diabetic care
4. Screening the elderly (i.e. the annual home visit)
In addition the practice nurse can expect to be increasingly involved
in the cervical cytology campaign (both in taking the smears and in
her health education role), the paediatric surveillance scheme and
the childhood immunization programme. She will also be assisting
the GP in minor surgery sessions. There may be considerable
overlap with the role of the district nurse.
  Note that GPs now have a responsibility for training their practice
nurses. For details of practice nurse training courses write to
English National Board for Nursing, Midwifery and Health Visiting,
Victory House, 170 Tottenham Court Road, London W1P 0HA

## The midwife
Their role includes a statutory duty to visit mothers daily for
10 days after delivery

## The health visitor
Health visitors have a broad job description and are expanding their
remit considerably in the field of preventative medicine. Much of
their workload is devoted to children but in some areas they are
able to concern themselves increasingly with the problems of the
elderly. Their responsibilities are:
1. Health education of mother and her new baby, giving advice on
   feeding and sleeping problems, crying babies, childhood
   illness and development. Visiting all children under 5 years is a
   statutory duty, the first visit usually being made after the
   midwife has left, i.e. after the tenth day
2. Further support and education of mothers at child health clinics
   and GPs' surgeries. They play a central role in the carrying out
   and assisting the doctor with development assessments and
   screening procedures (e.g. hearing tests)
3. Other preventative work, e.g. the immunization of children and
   work with the elderly
4. Surveillance of individuals at risk, e.g. single mothers, children
   at risk of abuse or the elderly living on their own
5. Mobilization of resources within the community – they are a
   mine of information on local support groups, mother-and-
   toddler groups, day nurseries, etc.

## The social worker
A social worker plays a particularly important role in the following
areas:
1. Counselling
   (i) Casework – helping individuals with their problems, be
       they personal, financial, marital or housing
   (ii) Formation and help with mutual support groups, e.g. for
       single mothers
   (iii) Marital counselling
2. The care of children
   (i) Work in child guidance clinics
   (ii) Supervision of children in care
   (iii) Monitoring and arranging adoption and fostering
   (iv) Support and counselling of disturbed children and their
       families
   (v) Liaison with day nurseries and vetting of childminders
   (vi) Involvement in many legal matters, notably in cases of
       child abuse with all the attendant legal procedures,
       registration, follow-up and, indeed, help and support to the
       families concerned

3. Mental health
   (i) Approved social workers play a part in compulsory admission to hospital under the Mental Health Act
   (ii) Follow-up and support of the mentally ill
4. Helping the elderly and disabled
   (i) Liaison with the hospital, occupational therapists, etc.
   (ii) Organizing transport, helping disabled people adapt and modify their homes, helping in the supply of aids to mobility
   (iii) Helping to provide home helps and meals-on-wheels
5. Housing and residential
   (i) Social workers are an important contact with the housing department
   (ii) Advice on legal rights, grants, etc.
   (iii) Help in finding accommodation
   (iv) Help, support and advice to homeless families
6. Mobilization of resources
   (i) A guide to the increasingly complex social security system, enabling the intimidated or bewildered to claim their full quota of benefits
   (ii) Mobilization of social support and financial benefits to those in need

## SPECIAL FEATURES OF GENERAL PRACTICE

### Appointments systems

*Advantages*
1. Convenience for the patient – with an appointment, should be able to avoid unnecessary waiting
2. Convenience for the GP – you can plan your week more effectively
3. Allows the practice to plan holidays and rotas to fit in with the surgery commitment
4. Allows a more even distribution of workload between the partners
5. Allows for planned and efficient use of the surgery, the reception staff and the nursing staff
6. Follow-up appointments for patients with chronic illness or hypertension can be easily arranged and you can structure the appointments to fit in with your own timetable
7. Special sessions (antenatal clinics, hypertension screening clinics, well baby clinics, etc.) can be organized so they do not clash with surgery time

*Disadvantages*
1. With an inflexible appointments system, patients with non-urgent problems may have to wait days to see a doctor

2. Appointments systems require more staff
3. Some patients may be discouraged from seeking medical attention by having to make an appointment
4. A few patients, chiefly the elderly, may not have a telephone or, indeed, friends or neighbours who can make an appointment for them
5. The local transport may not fit in with an appointments system, particularly in rural areas

## Rural practice

*Advantages*
1. Pleasant rural setting
2. You are the 'village GP'
3. Low list size with more time for each patient but with income at least partly maintained by dispensing and rural practice payments

*Disadvantages*
1. Travelling distance to visit patients
2. Isolation – colleagues/postgraduate centre/hospital may be miles away
3. Have to cope with emergencies with less hospital back-up
4. On-call – there may be little or no time off-duty

## Group practice
The advantages and disadvantages of group versus single-handed practice is summarized in Table 16

## Practice area
Areas are classified by list size thus:

|  | Average list size |
| --- | --- |
| Restricted area | 1700 or less |
| Intermediate area | 1701–2100 |
| Open area | 2101–2500 |
| Designated area | 2501+ |

GPs are paid a special allowance for practising in a designated area but they have now all but disappeared. There are still a dwindling number of open areas where you can start a practice by putting up your plate but the vast majority are classified as intermediate or restricted areas, where permission is required before a new GP can be appointed.

## The list size
1. The average list size in Britain currently stands at around the 1900 mark. The list size is highest in England and lowest in Scotland, with Wales and Northern Ireland in-between

**Table 16**

|  | Group practice | Single-handed practice |
|---|---|---|
| **1. Patient care** | | |
| Continuity of care | Can be a drawback, but personal lists can overcome this | Easier to control a patient'streatment and follow-up. Greater personal knowledge of patients |
| Choice | Patient has some choice | Patient has no choice |
| Skills | Partners possess different skills | |
| Visits | Availability, but may not be familiar with the patient, e.g. a large practice with a rota for out-of-hours cover | Familiar with patient, but may use deputizing, if available |
| List size | Can accommodate a large influx of new patients | May find it difficult to adapt to changes in the list size |
| **2. Night cover, weekend cover and holidays** | Rotas, hence adequate off-duty cover | May use deputizing but its use is being increasingly restricted. May be difficulty in finding locums |
| **3. Sickness** | Can cover for a partner when ill | Severe problems if sick. Need substantial insurance |
| **4. Premises** | Larger premises and can afford more expensive equipment | Smaller premises, usually with less equipment |
| **5. Attached staff** | May be a wide range – a full health care team | May be more limited and shared with other practices |
| **6. Decision-making** | Needs a consensus of opinion with good relationships and communication between partners | You alone decide |
| **7. Professional satisfaction** | Can discuss problems, clinical and non-clinical, with partners | A degree of professional isolation is inevitable |
| **8. Training and research** | Easier. Trainees benefit from seeing different partners at work. Research is easier with a larger list | Trainees may need some additional experience |

**Table 16**   (Contd)

|  | Group practice | Single-handed practice |
|---|---|---|
| 9. 1990 Contract screening and health promotion programmes | Easier to organize – more patients and GPs will have different expertise | Difficult to organize due to time and ? lack of expertise |
| 10. Business and financial aspects |  |  |
| Staff | May be many, hence organizational skills essential. A practice manager may help to maximize income | Few and hence easy to supervise, but staff costs may be proportionately greater |
| Running costs | Shared by partners |  |
| Dispensing | More profitable – can order in bulk, less stock per doctor, etc. |  |
| Deputizing service | May not need service in large groups or use it less |  |
| Outside appointments | Easier to take on |  |
| Recall schemes e.g. for cervical smears and immunizations | Possibility of large cost-effective schemes using computerized records and specially organized clinics |  |
| Holding a practice budget | Currently open to practices with lists of 5000+ | Cannot currently apply to hold a budget unless in combination with other practices |

2. The practice must define the geographical area from which it will accept patients. To register, a patient moving into the area presents his or her medical card to the practice or signs an FP1. The GP then signs the card, accepting the patient on his or her list
3. You can remove a patient from your list by writing to the FHSA, but 8 days elapse after the FHSA receives your request before the removal becomes effective

## INCOME

**Reference:** Statement of Fees and Allowances 1989
The main source of income is from the Health Authority and can be broken down into seven categories:
1. Capitation-based payments. These will make up over half (i.e. the majority) of Health Authority income. The income structure therefore strongly favours practices with a high list size
2. Allowances

3. Target payments for childhood immunization and cervical cytology
4. Item of service payments – now much reduced as a proportion of income. Still highly dependent on a young practice population (maternity, contraception, vaccinations not covered by the target scheme)
5. Sessional payments for minor surgery and teaching medical students
6. Other payments received by some practices but not others i.e. training, dispensing and rural practice payments
7. Health promotion payments

Other sources of income for a GP are:

1. Hospital work as a clinical assistant or hospital practitioner. GPs are also paid (from a bed fund) for covering GP cottage hospitals
2. Medical reports and examinations, e.g.
    (i) Life insurance medicals and reports
    (ii) Reports for solicitors
    (iii) Adoption and fostering medicals
    (iv) Examinations for attendance and mobility allowance
    (v) Heavy goods vehicle and elderly driver medicals
    (vi) Pre-employment medicals
3. Certificates, e.g.
    (i) Private certificates
    (ii) Cremation certificates
    (iii) Certificates for the notification of infectious diseases
4. Employment as a medical officer, e.g.
    (i) As a medical officer to a school
    (ii) As a medical officer to a factory or company on a part-time basis
5. Work as a police surgeon
6. Work as a member of a management team, medical board or tribunal
7. Work in local clinics, e.g. family planning clinics or child development clinics
8. Working sessions for the local deputizing service
9. Lecturing and writing
10. Private practice – but few GPs have more than a handful of private patients, if any, and there are restrictions placed on private practice if you wish to receive the full payments from the Health Authority
11. Miscellaneous, e.g. attending at a case conference or in court as a witness

**Capitation-based payments**
These are by far the most important source of income for a GP. The local Health Authority will send you your list size every quarter broken down into the following categories:

1. Patients aged 0–64 years
2. Patients aged 65–74 years
3. Patients aged 75 years and over
4. Temporary residents staying less than 15 days
5. Temporary residents staying more than 15 days

As from 1 May 1994 the annual fee received for a patient aged 0–64 is £14.60, for a patient aged 65–74 £19.30 and GPs will receive an annual payment of £37.30 for every patient aged 75 and over on their list (recognizing the work involved in screening, visiting and caring for the elderly).

The other capitation-based payments are:

1. Capitation fees for those children registered with a GP for the purpose of child health surveillance
2. Deprivation payments. These are additional payments for each patient who lives in a deprived area (the deprivation being judged in accordance with Professor Jarman's index of deprivation). There are three levels of payment – for patients living in high, medium and low areas of deprivation (defined respectively as areas with a score of over 50, 40–49 and 30–39 on the Jarman index)
3. Payments for the New Registration Check (see terms of service). A fee is payable if the New Registration Check is carried out within 3 months of the patient being accepted onto the list

**The main allowances from the Health Authority**
These form another appreciable portion of Health Authority income. There are three:

1. Basic Practice Allowance
   A payment based on partnership average list size. Payment starts at an average partnership list size of 400 and the maximum rate (£6816 from 1.4.94) will be given to those GPs with an average partnership list size of at least 1200 patients
2. Seniority Allowances
   These have now been effectively reduced by the PGEA (see below). There are three Seniority Allowances:
   (i) For allowance I you must have been registered for 11 years with 7 years as a GP
   (ii) For allowance II you must have been registered for 18 years with 14 years as a GP
   (iii) For allowance III you must have been registered for 25 years with 21 years as a GP
3. Postgraduate Education Allowance (PGEA)
   Paid for attending a programme of education consisting of 25 days over a 5-year period (i.e. 5 days a year), having attended over that time at least two courses from each of the following three categories:
   – Health promotion and prevention of illness

- Disease management
- Service management

Distance learning packages can also count towards qualification for the PGEA. The allowance has been set at a reasonable level (currently £2150) and all GPs will wish to qualify, although the course and subsistence fees will not be reimbursed – these must come out of the GP's pocket

**Target payments for childhood immunization and cervical cytology**
*See* relevant chapters

**Item of service payments**
The main ones are:
1. Maternity work – a complicated system of fees depending on when the patient books, responsibility or not for the confinement and whether the GP is on the obstetric list or not
2. Contraception – the ordinary fee for the pill, diaphragm and follow-up of patients with the coil is paid annually, assuming, of course you do the work and the patient signs the FP1001. There is a special fee for fitting an IUCD
3. Immunization – childhood immunization no longer appears here but GPs will still be paid for some travel immunizations, tetanus, etc.
4. Night visit fees – paid for visiting patients between the hours of 10 pm and 8 am. Currently a new system for rewarding night visits is being negotiated

*Health promotion payments*
Two categories of payment:
1. The banding system of payment. 3 bands:
   *Band 1*: Practices to construct an age – sex register, identify and counsel smokers (targeting priority groups)
   *Band 2*: Practices to set up a screening programme to identify patients aged 15–74 with hypertension. Registers to be constructed of those with hypertension, coronary heart disease and stroke. Must also fulfill band 1 requirements
   *Band 3*: Practices to set up a full coronary heart disease risk factor screening programme documenting the following on patients aged 15–74: smoking, blood pressure, family history, alcohol intake, diet, exercise and body mass index. Must also fulfill band 1 and 2 requirements
   Payments depend on list size and are heavily weighted towards band 3
2. Payments for having a diabetes care programme and/or an asthma care programme. These programmes should include:

- A register of asthmatics/diabetics
- A call/recall system
- Management plans for each patient
- Regular patient review, with the keeping of record cards
- Identification of criteria for hospital referral
- Adequate staff training
- Audit of the care provided

Payments are not dependant on list size

**Other major payments**
These include dispensing payments (*see* chapter on Prescribing),
training payments (the trainer being paid a training grant) and rural
practice payments (for practising in rural areas)

### EXPENDITURE, TAX AND ACCOUNTS

Inevitably there are expenses incurred in running a practice. They
can be subdivided into three groups, depending on the
reimbursement thus:
1. Expenses directly reimbursed by the Health Authority
     (i)  National Insurance contributions for the practice staff
     (ii) Rent of the premises (providing the district valuer agrees).
          If you own your own premises a 'notional' rent is paid
     (iii) Rates
2. Expenses partially reimbursed by the Health Authority
     A proportion of the salary of employed staff (providing those
     staff are properly qualified and trained). Health Authorities will
     enter into arrangements with GPs concerning the precise
     details and the arrangements will be subject to review
3. Expenses not reimbursed directly by the Health Authority
     (i)   Renewals, repairs and decoration of the premises
     (ii)  Telephone charges (including answering and paging
           services)
     (iii) Light and heat
     (iv)  Stationery, writing equipment and postage
     (v)   Insurance premiums
     (vi)  Accountancy and bank charges
     (vii) Dressings, equipment and drugs for the surgery
     (viii) The cost of using a deputizing service
     (ix)  Costs involved in cleaning the surgery
     (x)   A host of smaller 'miscellaneous' expenses

Group 3 expenses are taken into account when the Review
Body (the body determining GP's pay) reports each year. GP's
accounts and records are examined and an estimate made of
those practice expenses not directly reimbursed. This figure
(the 'indirect reimbursement of expenses') is added to what the
Review Body intends the average remuneration of a GP to be

for the coming year, e.g. currently the indirect reimbursement figure is £22 000 and the intended average remuneration of a GP for the year is £42 000, the Review Body having adjusted all the fees and allowances listed in the 'Income' section to yield a gross income for the average GP of £64 000

## Personal expenses
These include:
1. Motoring costs – running costs (petrol, services, repairs, tax, insurance) and an element for depreciation in the value of your car
2. Telephone charges
3. Professional subscriptions – GMC retention fee, MDU/MPS subscription, BMA, RCGP
4. Books, personal stationery, postage
5. Replacement of equipment
6. Spouse's salary and household expenses, as appropriate

## Income tax
GPs are self-employed and, as such, are taxed under schedule D. Tax is paid twice a year

## Pensions
Although self-employed GPs are also members of a superannuation scheme, contributing 6% of their superannuable income (income derived from the Health Authority with an amount deducted for expenses). The main entitlement is an index-linked annual pension of 1.4% of total superannuable earnings plus a tax-free lump sum of three times the annual pension.

## Accounts
What income is kept and what is divided between the partners differs from practice to practice and should be in the partnership contract. The practice's annual statement will list the income and expenditure thus:

*Practice income*
1. From FHSA allowances and fees
2. From other sources
3. Rent and rates reimbursement
4. Staff salaries reimbursement

*Practice expenditure*
1. Rent and rates (same figure as in income)
2. Staff salaries

3. Practice expenses (as in Group 3)
Practice net income = income – expenditure

To calculate your own income divide the practice net income by the number of partners (assuming all are on parity) or according to the agreed shares if not all on parity. You then deduct personal expenses and work out your tax on the remainder. The vast majority of practices employ an accountant to calculate all the necessary figures and tax. Since the above is but a brief summary and there are numerous intricacies in preparing practice accounts and negotiating with the Inland Revenue, it is a foolish economy to skimp on accountancy fees (themselves tax-allowable).

## VISITING

Most practices use a rota between the partners for out-of-hours calls. Visiting rates vary widely between practices and, indeed, between partners

### Principles of visiting

1. Educate patients how to request a visit – this information should be clearly set out in the practice booklet, including the procedure for night visits
2. Ensure the practice has efficient telephone answering/paging facilities so that visits can be quickly and reliably relayed to the partner on call
3. Make sure you personally
   (i) Have an efficient system for reviewing drugs and equipment in your bag for use in an emergency
   (ii) Have a working knowledge of the local geography
   (iii) Have your car serviced regularly and a second car available in the dire emergency of a breakdown
   (iv) Are familiar with the admission policies of the local hospitals
4. Construct an up-to-date list of all the telephone numbers you are likely to need in an emergency (social workers, night nurses, local pharmacies, partners and practice staff, ambulance service, etc.)
5. Obtain essential details first when a patient requests a visit, i.e.
   (i) Name of the patient
   (ii) Address to be visited
   (iii) Telephone number
   Then elicit the nature of the problem to assess:
   (i) The urgency of the visit
   (ii) Any drugs or equipment needed
   (iii) What advice you can offer prior to the visit

6. Decision to visit. While not legally required to visit at every request, 'failure to visit' appears commonly in the tales of medical disasters (and at service hearings) and you have to be on very firm ground in offering telephone advice rather than visiting even for seemingly innocuous requests. Certain visits are, of course, mandatory, e.g. chest pain. It is your responsibility to obtain the information necessary to make the decision about visiting – if in doubt, visit

## Arguments for and against using a deputizing service for out-of-hours call

*For*
1. If in a large group practice the patient may not see their own GP anyway
2. GPs need adequate rest and time off like anyone else, not least for their own family life
3. If called out at night the GP is likely to be less alert, communicative and efficient the next day
4. Finance. Night visit fees are still claimable on your behalf and use of a deputizing service is an allowable practice expense
5. In certain inner city areas it may be dangerous (especially for female GPs) to visit at night, whereas deputies have back-up from the driver, call systems, etc.
6. Deputizing services are, by and large, efficient. There is little evidence of excessive delay in answering urgent calls and the doctors employed are required to have GP experience – indeed many are local GPs doing sessions

*Against*
1. Patients generally prefer to see their own GP for out-of-hours calls
2. Deputizing services tend to visit for even the most trivial requests – this increases the visiting rate
3. The deputizing doctor has no personal knowledge of the patient and no ready access to the records. For the majority of calls this is, of course, unnecessary and in any case the GP can always be contacted
4. Cost – the cost depending on use. If you do your own night visits, you earn fees and do not have to pay a deputizing service
5. If a GP in a partnership has visited he or she can more easily discuss the visit and arrange appropriate follow-up the next day
6. Patients may be less inclined to call for a trivial reason if their own GP is on call, and if he or she were called they may be able

to offer simple advice (come round to the house later, pick up a prescription at the surgery, etc.)

Deputizing services are obviously features of urban conurbations rather than rural areas and their use by GPs is now restricted, the restrictions varying from area to area.

## PREMISES AND EQUIPMENT

### Health centres versus partnership-owned premises

*Advantages of health centres*
1. Little financial outlay – capital is provided by the Health Authority
2. May be spacious and well equipped with a high standard of fixtures and fittings and ample car parking space
3. Centralization of facilities – may be rooms for dietitians, physiotherapists, social workers, etc.
4. The Health Authority may employ some of the staff, relieving you of the tasks of working out salaries, etc.
5. Different practices in the same health centre may
   (i) Share resources to afford better equipment, e.g. telephone equipment, ECG, etc.
   (ii) Make the organizing of a special clinic a viable possibility, e.g. a clinic by a visiting consultant
   (iii) Make the organizing of postgraduate meetings at the health centre a useful venture
   (iv) With the increased number of patients, make research or other innovations easier
   (v) Share in an out-of-hours rota
6. In a health centre you may not need to worry so much about the cost of upkeep and repairs

*Advantages of partnership-owned premises*
1. Reimbursement by the Health Authority rent schemes means that owning a surgery is an excellent capital investment. There will be a substantial capital gain on retirement
2. Freedom to do what you wish with the premises – add to, convert, extend, change rooms, etc., (subject to reimbursement regulations)
3. Less restrictions on use, e.g. for private practice (need permission to see private patients in a health centre)
4. Having Health Authority employed staff can mean
   (i) Less flexibility (who works the bank holiday?)
   (ii) Difficulty in disciplining or dismissing staff
   (iii) A lack of a say in who is employed
5. May be friction and dispute between partnerships working from the same health centre

6. Independence and security of tenure – GPs in health centres have contracts with the Health Authority and a scenario could be envisaged where, because of this, their ability to practice could be curtailed
7. GPs in health centres are subject to a service charge (for heat, light, phones, etc.). With a large centre, used by many people, it is more difficult to control costs
8. In health centres with many paramedical staff, chiropodists, dietitians, etc., friction may develop regarding use of space, telephones, common rooms, etc.
9. May be petty rulings in health centres, e.g. over the size of desks, colour of the walls, etc., getting the Health Authority to fix repairs may be time-consuming

The *cost rent scheme* is a scheme designed to reimburse GPs for building a new surgery or converting an existing building to serve as a surgery. The *notional rent* is a rent paid to reimburse existing GPs for having their capital tied up in their own surgery. A new partner, on joining a practice who own their own premises, will be required to purchase a share in those premises. It may seem a daunting prospect but remember

1. It is a sound investment for the future
2. A loan can be arranged
3. You will benefit from the rent schemes in operation

The purchase of the premises is a vital area of the practice agreement.


## Equipment of a typical surgery

*General*
1. Telephone systems, answering machines, bleeps, patient call systems
2. Furniture – chairs, desks, filing cabinets, couches, etc.
3. Dictaphones and typewriters
4. Kitchen equipment and refrigerator
5. Waiting room chairs, tables, etc.
6. Storage space and cabinets for forms, stationery, prescriptions, etc.
7. Filing system for medical records
8. Library with books and journals
9. Security alarms
10. Cleaning equipment
11. Heating and lighting equipment in addition to that fixed to the premises
12. Treatment room equipment – speculae, surgical instruments, ear syringes, sutures, weighing scales, syringes and needles, sharps disposal bins, dressings, sterilizing unit, etc.
13. Doctor's own equipment – auriscope, stethoscope,

ophthalmoscope, proctoscope, patella hammer, measuring
tape, weighing scales, vision charts, peak flow meter,
sphygmomanometer, etc.

*Optional*
1. Photocopier
2. Computer – although now difficult to manage without one
3. Video equipment
4. Centrifuge

*Useful clinical equipment (worth purchasing)*
1. ECG
2. Haemoglobinometer
3. Glucometer
4. Cautery equipment (? including cryocautery equipment)
5. Microscope
6. Audiometer
7. Vitalograph
8. Incubator for urines
9. A practice nebulizer

*Note:* An area may be set aside for equipment required in
resuscitation (airways, adrenaline, etc.)

## TRAINING

To become a GP principal you must possess a Certificate of
Prescribed or Equivalent Experience issued by the Joint Committee
on Postgraduate Training for General Practice.* Following
registration you need to either join a 3-year vocational training
scheme or construct one of your own. One year is spent as a trainee
in general practice and 2 years in hospital posts, two of which
should be 6-month posts from an approved list (basically general
medicine, geriatrics, paediatrics, psychiatry, accident and
emergency, obstetrics or gynaecology).

### Ten aims of vocational training of the trainee
1. To motivate yourself for the future
2. To become proficient clinically in dealing with the wide range
   of conditions and problems presented to a GP
3. To develop a special interest in one or two areas of general
   practice
4. To qualify
   (i)  For the Family Planning Certificate
   (ii) For the Obstetric list
5. To past one or two examinations. The two of major importance

*JCPTGP, 14 Princes Gate, London SW7 1PU

are the DRCOG and the MRCGP but, with increasing interest in peadiatric care, the DCH would also be an advantage
6. To learn techniques in the hospital years, which will be useful in general practice (injecting joints, minor surgical procedures, etc.)
7. To become conversant with the ethics and protocol of being a GP
8. To familiarize yourself with the business side of general practice
9. To understand the responsibilities of a GP to his or her patients, staff and partners
10. To eventually obtain a satisfactory post as a general practice principal

**First steps in becoming a trainer**
1. Discussion of the prospects
   (i) With your partners
   (ii) With local trainers
   (iii) With the local course organizer, regional or associate adviser
2. Review of your clinical skills
   (i) By attending postgraduate meetings
   (ii) By considering the possibilities and setting up care programmes for hypertensives, diabetics and asthmatics within the practice
   (iii) By getting involved actively with the band 3 health promotion programme running in the practice
3. With regard to the practice
   (i) Ensure the medical records are satisfactory (letters and continuation cards in date order, summary cards and drug treatment cards for appropriate patients)
   (ii) Obtain a good selection of books for the practice library, e.g.
      a. *Tutorials in General Practice* Mead and Patterson, published by Churchill Livingstone
      b. *Research in General Practice* Howie, published by Croom Helm
      c. *Common diseases, their nature, incidence and care* Fry, published by MTP Press
      d. *Disease Data Book* Fry, published by MTP Press
      e. *Running a Practice* Jones et al, published by Croom Helm
   (iii) Provide a well-equipped trainee's room
   (iv) Acquire any equipment needed (ECG, glucometer, etc.)
   (v) Ensure the practice has a well-maintained age–sex register and disease registers
   (vi) Review the repeat prescribing system to ensure it is efficient and develop a method for looking at prescribing habits (? developing a prescribing policy/formulary for the practice)

4. Development of a special interest – this will be an attraction to a selection panel and is not an unreasonable expectation of a trainer
5. Audit and research – the trainer will be expected to have an idea of the principles of audit and research and will certainly be expected to encourage and supervise trainees doing projects. Read *Trainee Projects* (Occasional Paper 29 of the RCGP)
6. Consider how the practice can adapt itself successfully to the New Contract and the prospect of holding a fund (if this is thought desirable)
7. Review the practice's computer system – computerization will figure so prominently in the general practice of the future that a good case can be made for computerizing all training practices

**Criteria for trainer selection**
The appointments are made by the General Practice Subcommittee of the Regional Postgraduate Medical Education Committee. The JCPTGP's criteria (reproduced with permission) include:
1. Evaluation of the trainer's personal characteristics
   (i) His or her availability
   (ii) His or her clinical competence (as judged by local reputation, involvement in local educational programmes, postgraduate diplomas – especially the MRCGP, etc.)
   (iii) His or her commitment to continuing medical education, including attendance at trainers' workshops and a willingness to subject themselves to performance review
   (iv) His or her ability to communicate
2. Evaluation of the trainer's teaching ability
   (i) His or her preparation for teaching
   (ii) His or her enthusiasm and commitment to teaching
   (iii) His or her skills as a teacher
3. Evaluation of the teaching practice
   Minimum educational criteria for training practices appear below (i)-(v) (reproduced with permission from the 1986 RCGP Members Reference Book, page 252, from an article by Dr Bill Styles. Publishers are Sterling Publications)
   (i) All medical records and hospital correspondence must be filed in date order
   (ii) Appropriate medical records must contain easily discernible drug therapy lists for patients on long-term therapy
   (iii) Practices should be starting to create summary problem lists where they do not exist
   (iv) Training practices should be developing methods for monitoring prescribing habits as an important part of the audit process
   (v) All training practices should have a library containing a selection of books and journals relevant to general practice

In addition to the above, premises must be adequate, equipment available, regular contact with members of the health care team possible and supervised experience of out-of-hours calls should be obtainable. On a wider front, the JCPTGP places considerable emphasis on prevention (including developmental surveillance), screening programmes and the care of patients with chronic diseases. Age – sex registers and disease registers are encouraged

## APPLYING FOR A PARTNERSHIP

1. Find out as much as you can about the partnership, especially
    (i) Locality
    (ii) Number, sex and age of the partners
    (iii) Health centre or privately owned premises
    (iv) Special interests or features of the practice, e.g. dispensing, training, etc.
    (v) Reasons for the partnership vacancy, e.g. retirement, expansion, etc.
2. With some practices it would help to have some informal contact prior to the official interviews but this may also irritate if there are a large number of applicants. The enthusiasm to visit the area informally, see the surgery and assess the local housing would, however, be noted
3. Curriculum vitae
    (i) Must be professionally typed with a handwritten cover note
    (ii) Explain why you wish to join this particular practice – singling out special areas where your interests coincide and you can be of particular help, e.g. obstetric work in a local maternity home, paediatric developmental clinics, minor surgery, etc.
    (iii) Structure your curriculum vitae as shown in Table 17
    *Notes on the c.v.:*
        a. Qualifications – DRCOG is a definite plus. If you have not been fortunate enough to have completed a 6-months post in obstetrics make absolutely sure that you obtain sufficient experience to be eligible for the obstetric list. Make sure too that you point out your eligibility as this is an essential requirement for most practices and your c.v. will fail without it. Paediatric experience (in view of the payment system for child health surveillance) is now also very important. The Family Planning Certificate is useful and many practices will expect you to be sitting the MRCGP
        b. Education – opposite the entries list any honours, distinctions or additional qualifications
        c. 'During vocational training' and 'special interests' – a chance in both to distinguish your application from the

**Table 17**    Specimen curriculum vitae

| | |
|---|---|
| NAME: J.B. | AGE: 30 |
| ADDRESS: | |
| NATIONALITY: | TELEPHONE NUMBER: |
| MARITAL STATUS: | e.g. married to a nurse and we have two children |
| QUALIFICATIONS: | e.g. MB BS DCH |

            Sitting DRCOG in April 1995
            Sitting MRCGP in October 1995
            Family Planning Certificate

EDUCATION:      e.g.
19–19 Attended XXX School
19–19 Entered XXX Medical School
            Qualified in MB BS with Honours in
            Pathology
19–19 Pre-registration House Surgeon to Dr X at
            XXX Hospital
19–19 Pre-registration House Physician to Prof X at
            XXX Hospital
19–19 Joined the XXX Vocational Training Scheme
            have completed the following posts
            SHO Obstetrics.....6 months
            SHO Geriatrics......6 months
            SHO Medicine........6 months
            SHO Paediatrics....6 months

CURRENT POSITION:  Trainee to Dr Kind,
                      Pleasant Health Centre,
                      Leafy Suburb,
                      Averagetown

During vocational training I sat on...(list committees sat on, research projects undertaken, prizes won, i.e. anything of interest that stands you out from the crowd)

| | |
|---|---|
| SPECIAL INTERESTS: | A chance here to demonstrate your value to this particular practice, e.g. 'I am especially interested in maternity work and note with enthusiasm that practice has deliveries in a local GP maternity unit.' |
| HOBBIES: | Helps to complete the picture of you as an individual |
| AVAILABILITY: | Make sure you can start when they want you to |

GMC REGISTRATION NUMBER:
MDU/MPS MEMBERSHIP:
CURRENT DRIVING LICENCE and I own a XXX car

others. If you have other unusual features in your past history, e.g. a year in Africa or a leading article in the BMJ, mention them. Alternatively, 10 years as a surgical registrar in Iceland may be less of a plus point on the c.v.

   d. Hobbies – again if you are the county squash captain
       mention it
   e. GMC registration/defence union/driving licence – all
       show a practical knowledge of what is required
*Note:* The handwritten cover note is just as important as the c.v. in
distinguishing you as an enthusiastic, literate individual with one or
two intriguing characteristics (but not too way out!)

**Tips for the interview**
1. Arrive smartly dressed at the correct time
2. Be natural and do not pretend to be something you are not
3. Do not be too keen to discuss money matters – this will come
   later
4. Remember the interview may be your only chance to assess
   the practice – make a mental note of what you wish to know
   about the practice and its future development
5. Your spouse should accompany you to the interview – she or he
   will inevitably be involved with the practice in some way and
   will also need to assess housing, schools, etc.
6. Try during the interview to assess the philosophy and
   motivations of the practice and where they see themselves
   heading in the future.
       Before deciding to join the partnership, two general rules:
   (i) Do not be put off by having to buy into a practice – it is an
       excellent investment
   (ii) Join a practice without a partnership agreement at your
       peril. The partnership agreement should cover all the main
       areas of practice (retirement, distribution of income,
       premises, expulsion, illness, etc.)

**CERTIFICATION**

**Sickness certification**

*Self-certification*
Used for periods of inability to work for 7 days or less – no need to
see the GP unless requiring treatment. Also used for the first 7 days
of a longer illness

*Notes on Form Med 3 (the white 'sick certificate')*
1. Must be written and signed in indelible ink, the patient seen
   and the certificate given 'no later than the day after the
   examination to which it relates'
2. First decision is the length of time the patient should refrain
   from work. You can issue a 'closed' certificate, i.e. filling in a
   specific date to return to work, if it is estimated that the patient
   can return to work within 2 weeks

3. If the patient cannot return to work within 2 weeks you must issue an open statement. Open statements can be up to 6 months but clearly if the patient is ill enough to need long-term sickness certification he or she will need to be reviewed
4. If you issue an open statement then, when the patient becomes fit enough to work again, you must issue a closed statement to return to work
5. After the patient has been off work with an open statement for 6 months you can, if it's unlikely the patient will work for a long time, fill in after 'until' the words 'further notice'
6. Diagnosis of the disorder. GPs are asked to be as precise as possible (fractured femur rather than leg injury) to assist in the collection of statistics. If you feel the patient should not know the precise diagnosis, fill in a vague diagnosis on Form Med 3 and send the correct diagnosis to the Regional Medical Officer on Form Med 6 (saves the patient being called for an RMO medical)
7. Should you wish a second opinion on the patient's ability to work, you can refer for an RMO opinion by filling in Form RM7
8. If the patient loses a certificate another can be issued with 'DUPLICATE' written on the top
9. Keep sickness certificates under lock and key as security stationery

*Note on Form Med 5 (the pink 'special statement')*
Used when the patient is not seen but you have received a written report issued less than 1 month previously satisfying you that the patient will not be able to work

**Medical certificates of the cause of death**
The following should be reported to the coroner:
1. Death where the cause is unknown or an unnatural cause is suspected
2. Death due to neglect, starvation, violence or an accident (e.g. a road traffic accident)
3. Death due to an industrial disease (a list of some of the common diseases of industrial origin appears on the back of the death certificate)
4. Death during an operation or before recovery from the anaesthetic
5. Death due to an abortion
6. Death as a result of medication, drugs or poisons
7. Suicide
8. Death due to 'injury' – including burns, suffocation, drowning, hypothermia, wounds and fractures. Tetanus is also to be reported
9. Death of the newborn, due to injury

10. Serum hepatitis (hepatitis B) or 'viral hepatitis'
11. Where the patient was not attended during his or her last illness by a medical practitioner
12. Where the patient had not been seen within 14 days of death. Failure to have seen the patient within 14 days before death is the commonest cause to be reported to the coroner in general practice

*Certifying the cause of death*
Solely indicating the mode of dying (cardiac failure, cardiac arrest) is not allowed – you must on the certificate specify the underlying disease (myocardial infarction, carcinomatosis due to carcinoma of the bronchus, etc.)

**The cremation forms**
B (Part 1) – the doctor must have been in attendance before death and have seen the body after death
C (Part 2) – the doctor must have been registered (not just qualified) for 5 years and must not be a relative or partner of the doctor who has signed the first part

**POLITICS**
1. British Medical Association
     (i)   The professional association of doctors in this country
    (ii)   Has a partnership introduction and locum service
   (iii)   Can give advice and help on a wide range of matters (partnership agreements, employment, taxation, superannuation, ethics, legal matters)
    (iv)   Publishes the British Medical Journal
2. Local Medical Committee (LMC)
     (i)   A group of local GPs, elected by local GPs
    (ii)   Each GP pays a levy to finance the LMC
   (iii)   Negotiates with and advises the local Health Authority
    (iv)   Representatives help individual GPs with problems (e.g. complaints, illness, terms of service, etc.)
3. General Medical Services Committee (GMSC)
   A committee of the BMA negotiating with the DHSS on the terms and conditions of service for all general practitioners
4. Joint Committee on Postgraduate Training for General Practice (JCPTGP)
   Supervises vocational training and issues the necessary certificates (*see* section on Training)
5. Royal College of General Practitioners
     (i)   National organization divided throughout the country into faculties
    (ii)   Membership by examination twice a year

(iii)  Trainees can become associate members
(iv)  Concerned with continuing education, performance review and research. Provides information services for GPs. Publishes reports, occasional papers and the Journal of the RCGP. Runs the MRCGP examination. The central headquarters in London houses a large reference library
6.  Young principal groups
   (i)  Maintain the enthusiasm engendered by vocational training
  (ii)  Main functions support and intellectual stimulation

*Note:* Trainees can participate in all the above (except obviously young principal groups), both locally and nationally. In particular, there are trainee observers on the RCGP, JCPTGP and on a special trainees subcommittee of the GMSC

## CONFIDENTIALITY AND ETHICS

### Confidentiality
Consultations between GP and patient should be strictly confidential. Disclosure of confidential information by the GP is a serious breach of ethics. You can, of course, discuss matters with your partners and other members of the health care team but anyone to whom confidential information is given must also appreciate the ethics of confidentiality. Only rarely will disclosure be judged to be in the public interest – consult your defence society before any disclosure to a third party without written consent from the patient. This ruling does not, of course, apply to the reporting of official statistics and notifications, e.g. of infectious diseases. The commonest difficulties in general practice concern driving, e.g. a newly diagnosed epileptic. Prescribing contraception is another thorny issue.

### Code of ethics
Best learnt by example. The BMA publish *The Handbook of Medical Ethics*, which is worth reading

### Medical defence
It is essential that every GP is a member of a medical defence society, e.g. the Medical Defence Union or the Medical Protection Society and compulsory membership of a defence society is usually written into the partnership contract. Reading their annual reports is instructive. Certain clinical problems are renowned for litigation – foreign bodies in the eye, missed fractured scaphoid, etc.

# Prescribing

## NOTES ON THE USE OF THE FP10 (THE 'PRESCRIPTION') AND GENERAL NOTES ON PRESCRIBING

1. An FP10 is valid for 13 weeks from the date it is signed
2. At the top of the FP10 is a space for age if under 12 years
3. The letters NP (Nomen Propium) near the top of the FP10 mean the drug dispensed will be labelled with the name of the prescribed drug. If you do not wish the name of the prescribed drug to appear you can delete the letters NP
4. If you fill in the number of days treatment, e.g. 30, then, providing you indicate the dosage and frequency of use, the pharmacist will dispense the precise quantity of drug. If you do not fill in the number of days treatment then you must specify the quantity of each drug to be dispensed along with the dose and frequency of use

## ACBS

There are borderline substances which can only be prescribed in certain situations, e.g. gluten-free products for those with coeliac disease or Wysoy for babies with lactose intolerance. If not prescribed for this specific reason payment will be withheld for your error. When prescribing a borderline substance for a permitted indication write 'ACBS' (Advisory Committee on Borderline Substances) next to the prescribed product – the prescription will then normally pass through with no payment deducted

## GENERIC PRESCRIBING

We are encouraged to prescribe generically (i.e. frusemide rather than Lasix) but there are also arguments against (bioavailability, presentation, etc.)

## THE LIMITED LIST

We are now limited in certain areas of prescribing, e.g.

tranquillizers, cough mixtures, analgesics, antacids and laxatives. If a blacklisted preparation (i.e. not available at NHS expense) is required for a patient (e.g. Frisium, Dalmane, etc.) then a private prescription must be issued. Note that Frisium can be prescribed for epileptics if the FP10 is endorsed 'S3B'

## INDICATIVE PRESCRIBING BUDGETS

Since 1 April 1991 GPs have been subject to the 'indicative prescribing scheme'. Note, however, that fundholders will have prescribing costs included with their general fund. The indicative prescribing scheme works as follows:

1. The Health Authority allocates the practice an amount to cover its prescribing costs. The Health Authority will take into account the current prescribing pattern of the practice, the average prescribing costs in the area and any special factors relevant to the practice (e.g. a few patients on very expensive medication)
2. Every month the practice receives from the Prescription Pricing Authority, a statement of the amount spent by the practice on prescribing and this will be a way of monitoring how your expenditure is matching the allocation of funds
3. At the end of the financial year the Health Authority will examine the practice's prescribing expenditure. If the practice has exceeded the allocated amount there are several possibilities viz:
   (i) After explanation from the practice, the Health Authority may accept that the increased expenditure was justified on the basis of patient need
   (ii) If the Health Authority considers the prescribing to be excessive without clinical justification, it can refer the GP(s) to a hearing in front of a committee of three doctors and this may result in the withholding of income from those GP(s)
4. Each Health Authority will appoint a medical adviser to liaise with practices where prescribing is deemed to be a problem (this includes under-prescribing as well as over-prescribing)
5. Practice formularies are to be encouraged but not compulsory

### REFERENCE

Improving Prescribing. Department of Health 1990

## CONTROLLED DRUGS

Controlled drugs (preceded by CD in the National Formulary or MIMS) are a special category in that the prescription must be written in ink (or otherwise as to be indelible) in the prescriber's own handwritting and must include:

1. The name and address of the patient
2. The form, strength and dose of the preparation and the frequency with which the dose should be taken
3. The total quantity of drug to be dispensed in words and figures
4. The doctor's signature and date
5. The address of the doctor

The controlled drugs to which the above regulations apply include:

barbiturates
buprenorphine (Temgesic)
dextromoramide (Palfium)
diamorphine
Diconal
diethylpropion (Tenuate Dospan)
dihydrocodeine by injection

methadone (Physeptone)
morphine in its various forms
pentazocine (Fortral, Fortagesic)
pethidine

So-called 'schedule 2' drugs (including morphine, diamorphine and pethidine) must be kept under lock and key. You must keep a record of the controlled drugs you personally administer. This is one area of concern to the Regional Medical Officer

## ADDICTS

GPs are required to notify suspected addicts to the Chief Medical Officer – see the British National Formulary for details. It is illegal for general practitioners to prescribe diamorphine, Diconal or cocaine to addicts without a special licence

*Notes:*
1. Prescription pads must be securely locked away and prescriptions should not be left for collection in an unsupervised situation. Do not sign a blank prescription
2. Obvious drugs of addiction are pethidine, dextromoramide, etc., but patients can also become dependent on a much wider range of drugs. Keep a check on repeat prescriptions, requests for benzodiazepines, etc.

## PRESCRIPTION CHARGES

Prescriptions are free for
1. Children under 16 years (and over 16 years if still at school)
2. Women aged 60 years and over
3. Men aged 65 years and over
4. Pregnant women (and up to 1 year after birth)
5. Patients with low incomes and War or Service pensioners (see DHSS leaflets)
6. Patients with a fistula, diabetes mellitus, epilepsy requiring continuous anticonvulsants, myxoedema and a few other disorders requiring 'replacement' medication

Prescriptions are not free for hypertensives, asthmatics, those with arthritis, etc., and these groups may wish to purchase a 'season ticket'

## ADVERSE REACTIONS – THE 'YELLOW CARD' SYSTEM

The Committee on Safety of Medicines relies on doctors to report any suspected adverse reactions to them using the 'yellow cards'. This especially applies to newer agents (marked ▼ in MIMS)

## DISPENSING

*Dispensing doctors* are paid for dispensing drugs via a complicated drug tariff system (the alternative capitation system having ceased). The fee for a prescription is currently worked out as:
Basic drug price + 10.5%
+
A container allowance
+
A dispensing fee, which reduces the more prescriptions per month dispensed
+
A VAT allowance
Reducing the payment made to the doctor is a discount scale on the basic drug price
*Non-dispensing doctors* may still buy in and administer certain drugs to patients (notably injections, IUCDs and sutures) and claim on the above system by submitting the relevant FP10s to the Prescription Pricing Authority by the fifth day of the following month. Apart from injections of emergency drugs, vaccinations and steroid-containing injections (e.g. Depo-Medrone) are common examples of drugs that can be 'dispensed' by non-dispensing doctors

## DRUGS FOR THE GP's BAG

The following would be the contents of a typical GP's drugs bag

**Drugs for oral use**

| | |
|---|---|
| Antibiotics: | Amoxycillin (+sachets for children) |
| | Penicillin |
| | Erythromycin(+Erythroped for children) |
| | Flucloxacillin |
| Analgesics: | Paracetamol |
| | Dihydrocodeine |
| | Naproxen |
| Bronchodilator: | Salbutamol tablets |

| | |
|---|---|
| Antihistamines | Chlorpheniramine (Piriton) |
| | Terfenadine (Triludan) |
| Diuretic: | Frusemide |
| Tranquillizer: | Diazepam (2 mg and 5 mg) |
| | Chlordiazepoxide |
| | Chlorpromazine |
| Antidiarrhoeal: | Imodium capsules |
| | Dioralyte sachets (for children) |
| Steroids: | EC Prednisolone 5 mg |
| Antacid: | Gaviscon tablets |
| Anti-emetics: | Prochlorperazine (Stemetil) |
| Cardiac: | Glyceryl trinitrate spray |
| | Sorbichew |
| | Digoxin 0.0625 mg and 0.125 mg |
| | Aspirin! |

**Suppositories**
Prochlorperazine (Stemetil)
Bisacodyl or other laxative

**Eye drops**
Fluorescein (for diagnosis)
Chloramphenicol

**Inhaler**
Ventolin or Bricanyl (plus Nebuhaler/Volumatic)
Access to a nebulizer useful

**Drugs by injection**
Adrenaline
Aminophylline
Amoxycillin
Atropine
Benzylpenicillin
Chlorpheniramine (Piriton)
Chlorpromazine (Largactil)
Cyclimorph or Diamorphine
Diazepam (Valium)
Diclofenac (Voltarol)
Dihydrocodeine
Frusemide (Lasix)
Glucagon
Glucose for i.v. injection (but Glucagon more useful)
Hydrocortisone
Naloxone
Pethidine – although many now use diclofenac for renal colic
Prochlorperazine (Stemetil)

Promazine (Sparine)
Salbutamol (Ventolin)
Syntometrine
Triplopen

**Other items apart from stationery**
Stesolid applicators – diazepam 5 mg for rectal use
Dextrostix/BM Stix
Clinistix
Silk/catgut, etc., for suturing
Emergency equipment may also be kept with the drugs bag, e.g.
airways, cannulas, etc.

**Notes**
1. Remember to stock a good supply of water for injection, syringes and needles
2. Check periodically that the drugs are not past the expiry date
3. Keep a special book to list the controlled drugs
4. Particularly important are adrenaline for anaphylaxis, diazepam for convulsions (including Stesolid for rectal use in children), glucagon for hypoglycaemia in diabetics, and i.v. hydrocortisone and salbutamol for use in patients with severe asthma. Frusemide for cardiac failure is essential and for renal colic, acute gout, backache or severe sprains seen on a home visit an injection of Voltarol is highly effective (assuming no history of peptic ulceration or drug-induced asthma attacks). Remember aspirin for suspected myocardial infarcts
5. Many GPs use a separate drugs bag for the above and a second bag for essential forms (prescriptions, sickness certificates, notepaper, continuation cards, temporary resident forms, etc.) and equipment (stethoscope, auriscope, ophthalmoscope, sphygmomanometer, thermometer, gloves, airway, etc.). How much extra equipment is carried for emergencies (nasal packing equipment, resuscitation equipment, obstetric equipment, etc.) depends on the expertise of the GP, the nearness or otherwise of the local Casualty and the special features and situation of the GP's practice

## REPEAT PRESCRIPTIONS

1. Each practice has its own system, repeat cards being kept by the patient. Each repeat card should ideally have recorded the drugs, dosages, frequency of use, quantities to be dispensed, date of issue of the repeat card and a review date. The current treatment regime should also be recorded on a card in the medical records

2. Each time a prescription is issued it should be recorded in the medical records so that a check can be kept on patient usage
3. Repeat prescriptions are customarily given for 1 or 2 months supply of medication
4. There should be an efficient system for review (e.g. by having a review date or expiry date on the repeat card)
5. Many practices are computerizing their repeat prescription system but keep up to date and remember prescriptions for controlled drugs have to be written by hand
6. Check repeat prescriptions carefully before signing them – you are legally responsible regardless of who has actually filled the prescription in
7. It has been estimated that about half of all prescriptions are written without actually seeing the patient, i.e. chiefly repeat prescriptions

# References

Allum W H, Hallissey M T, Dorrell A, Low J, Fielding J W L 1986 Programme for early detection of gastric cancer. British Medical Journal 293:541

Amery A et al 1985 Mortality and morbidity results from the European Working Party on High Blood Pressure in the Elderly trial. Lancet i:1349

Bain D J G 1983 Can the clinical course of acute otitis media be modified by systemic decongestant or antihistamine treatment? British Medical Journal 287:654

Bain J, Murphy E, Ross F 1985 Acute otitis media: clinical course among children who received a short course of high dose antibiotic. British Medical Journal 291:1243

Jones R, Bain J 1986 Three-day and seven-day treatment in acute otitis media: a double-blind antibiotic trial. Journal of the Royal College of General Practitioners 36:356

Kay E, Bailie G 1989 New drugs for urinary tract infections. Update 39:421

Lightowler C D R 1984 Injuries to the lateral ligament of the ankle. British Medical Journal 289:1247

Medical Research Council Working Party 1985 MRC trial of treatment of mild hypertension: principal results. British Medical Journal 291:97

RCGP 1986 Alcohol – a balanced view. Report from General Practice 24

Shapiro S 1977 Evidence on screening for breast cancer from a randomized trial. Cancer 39:2772

UK National Case – Control Study Group 1989 Oral Contraceptive use and breast cancer in young women. Lancet i:973

Valdini A 1985 Fatigue of unknown aetiology — a review. Family Practice 2 (1):48

# Index